Sexual Grounding Therapy

This important book explores the history of sexuality and the breadth of support available to people experiencing sex and relationship challenges, presenting a model of psychosexual therapy that's contextualised in the past, present and future and examined within a developmental and relational framework.

Sexual Grounding Therapy focusses on the work of Willem Poppeliers, who developed his unique approach to sex and relationship issues in the 1990s. Geoff Lamb explores the model's historical context; offers a comparison with other contemporary approaches, both mainstream and alternative; describes the model and its application in detail; and looks at future directions for this innovative work. While Poppeliers' approach to psychosexual therapy is radical, Geoff's book emphasises and goes beyond this, taking a controversial stance on such topics as sexuality and religion, psychotherapy and science, and the position of both psychotherapy and psychosexual therapy in today's society.

Sexual Grounding Therapy explores how people's needs at each stage of their lifelong psychosexual development relate to any current sex and relationship problems they may be experiencing. It will be invaluable, not only to professionals – counsellors, psychotherapists and others whose work involves sex and relationships – but also to readers who are interested in exploring their own self-development and relationships from a historical, social and family perspective.

Geoff Lamb has been a practising psychotherapist for 35 years. He also practises as a couple and psychosexual therapist. Geoff retired as director of the counselling training institute, Inter-Psyche, in 2017 and, apart from his practice, his spare time is now spent writing/reviewing, choral singing, gardening and spending time with his wife and grown-up family.

"The title of this book says it all – as individuals, and as a society, there is an urgent need to become grounded in our sexual understanding and expression for the overall health of humanity. Extremely well written and researched, *Sexual Grounding Therapy* is a valuable resource, especially for therapists and professionals working on the subject of sexuality and its expression in relationships. It clearly establishes the significance of addressing sex in a grounded and direct way."

Diana Richardson, author of several books on sex, including the best-seller, *The Heart of Tantric Sex*

Sexual Grounding Therapy

Context, Theory and Practice

Geoff Lamb

Routledge
Taylor & Francis Group

LONDON AND NEW YORK

First published 2021
by Routledge
2 Park Square, Milton Park, Abingdon, Oxon OX14 4RN

and by Routledge
605 Third Avenue, New York, NY 10158

Routledge is an imprint of the Taylor & Francis Group, an informa business

© 2021 Geoff Lamb

British Library Cataloguing-in-Publication Data
A catalogue record for this book is available from the British Library

Library of Congress Cataloging-in-Publication Data
A catalog record has been requested for this book

ISBN: 978-0-367-76394-7 (hbk)
ISBN: 978-0-367-86257-2 (pbk)
ISBN: 978-1-003-16676-4 (ebk)

Typeset in Bembo
by Taylor & Francis Books

This book is dedicated to Willem Poppeliers.
The modest, inspired genius who the created the work that forms its subject matter.

Contents

Figures

Acknowledgements

In the process of writing this book I am grateful to:

Helena Løvendal, for believing in me.

Véro/Vasanti, for her support and especially for her challenge along the way.

Ingo, for being my therapeutic brother and a challenging/supportive colleague.

Jane, for being my beautiful life partner, for her patience during the writing of this book and for her excellent proofreading.

Jonathan, my son, for the diagrams and the book cover.

Becca, my daughter, for reading the manuscript and for some challenging discussions about the content.

My colleagues, whose names are mentioned in the text, for their contributions and reviews of specific content.

Preface

This book represents, for me, a significant staging post on the journey that Sexual Grounding has become in my life. I first encountered this work in 2006 when it was recommended to me by Helena Løvendal and Nick Duffell. It came along at exactly the right time in my life – a year earlier and I would have dismissed it as 'a nice idea, but not for people like me', i.e., for people with a lot more money (I was between jobs for most of 2005)! A year later and I might already have committed myself to something like a professional doctorate or to some other form of advanced training.

The Sexual Grounding Therapy (SGT) model is also, as this book will show, a timely arrival in a world where, although we are no longer hidebound by the restrictions on talking and writing about sexuality, the quest for a fulfilling and intimate sexual relationship still represents an elusive challenge to many of us. This is reflected both in the relationships I encounter in my couplework practice and in newspaper articles such as that by Nicola Davies (Davies, 2020) headlined 'Half of British women have "poor sexual health"'.

When I went on my first Sexual Grounding Therapy workshop in Le Hammeau des Étoiles (a residential centre near Montpellier), I'd already undertaken countless hours of individual and group therapy and trained in Reichian Bioenergetic work and couples' counselling. I was certainly not a novice, but I realised that this work had something to offer me as far as my personal (and professional) development was concerned. However, in acknowledging the impact of Sexual Grounding Therapy, it is not my intention to dismiss my previous therapeutic experience – I don't think therapy works like that. Every therapist I have seen and every workshop or group I've attended seems to have built on the one before, and, had I not had this experience, I don't believe I would have gained so much from SGT.

Without going into my experience of it in detail, I would say that Sexual Grounding Therapy enabled me to 'rewrite my story' in a way that developed my previous therapeutic experience and harmonised with it both on a personal and professional level. In embarking on this book and the thesis that has provided the basis for it, my aim has been to put Sexual Grounding Therapy into the context of its historical development, present context and future perspective.

In the process of writing it, I realise that the other context I've put the work into is my own life journey as a psychotherapist.

Even though, as will become clear in the following pages, it is a development of the original model of psychotherapy developed by Freud, Sexual Grounding Therapy is nevertheless challenging and controversial, as indeed Freud's work was when it emerged towards the end of the 19th century. The challenging and controversial nature of psychotherapeutic approaches and how this is either eroded or maintains its sharpness will be explored at various points in the book.

Most books on psychotherapy and personal growth seem to assume a universal applicability. This book *doesn't*. Even those books which are aimed at specific 'problem areas' make the assumption that their model will work universally across that area. I don't do this. I'm writing about Sexual Grounding Therapy because it worked for *me*, so much so that I decided to train in the model.[1] In this way, I don't believe I'm doing anything different from many other writers/practitioners who write about their own or a colleague's work.[2] I've also seen great transformation in some of the SGT participants whose process I've been privileged to witness over the years. But I don't believe that one model or style of therapy works for everyone or that any one model of therapy will solve all of a person's issues, and I'm not aiming to persuade the reader that SGT is the exception.

Having established this limitation, I have now given myself the freedom to write passionately about my thoughts and beliefs, not only about this exciting development in the field of psychosexual therapy but also about the world in which it was created and is now practised. I'd like to invite the reader to take in, and benefit from, whatever 'speaks to' them, to give some thought to ideas they may find challenging and to let go of anything that, for whatever reason, they really find indigestible. My intent in writing this book is serious, but I don't take its contents, or myself, that seriously. Neither should you.

I'm aware that readers will be drawn to this book for different reasons and with different needs. I've structured it in a way that makes sense to me, setting the scene by giving the historical and contemporary context, then going on to explore the theory and practice of Sexual Grounding Therapy and finally looking into the future context. However, if what *you* want is to learn about the theory and practice first and then find out more about the historical and contemporary context you could just as easily start with Part 3 and move on to the other parts in whatever order seems logical to you.

Finally, I'm assuming that, as I do when I read, many readers will be either consciously or unconsciously self-reflecting as they read, asking themselves, 'How does this apply to or fit with my life experience?' To facilitate this, I have included one or two experiential/self-reflective exercises, which I hope will help readers to make personal sense of specific aspects of the work.

Notes

1 This is the way I've approached all of my psychotherapy training, although I recognise that I may be out of step with the current approach to psychotherapy and counselling training in doing it this way. As someone who has been involved in training counsellors for most of my professional life, I have to say I would have been glad if some of my students had taken this approach rather than undertaking the therapy just because it was a training requirement. This is partly because I believe that undertaking the therapy because you recognise the value of it in your own life will ultimately make you a better therapist and partly because it's easier to learn the theory and skills of therapy from the inside than from the outside – in other words it would have made my job as a trainer easier!

2 It has been argued that most originators of psychotherapeutic models do so as a result of, perhaps even as a way of, overcoming their own psychological difficulties. I see this as a strength rather than a criticism.

Reference

Davies, N. (2020). Half of British women 'have poor sexual health'. *The Guardian*, 9 January 2020.

Introduction

The year in which I wrote the thesis on which this book is based was the 25th anniversary of Willem Poppeliers' development of his unique model of body psychotherapy, Sexual Grounding Therapy (SGT). I found it surprising that so little had been written about this powerful and controversial psychotherapeutic method, and this motivated both my thesis and this book.

There are a number of short articles on SGT, both by Poppeliers himself and by his initial cohort of trainees (N. Fischer, 2002; Duffell & Poppeliers, 2006), and a short book that Poppeliers wrote in collaboration with the Dutch journalist Martin Broesterhuizen (Poppeliers & Broesterhuizen, 2007).[1] The emphasis in all of these is on summarising the SGT model and giving some information about its application in practice. This is undoubtedly useful, but what seems to me to be missing is a clear idea of where the model comes from, how it developed and where its roots are.

Similarly, it's difficult for the reader to get a good sense of where SGT locates itself in relation to other psychotherapeutic models. Some progress in this direction has been made by Notburga Fischer (2002) who, in her article, makes links between Sexual Grounding and her other therapeutic influences, and the book *Sexual Grounding Therapy* (Poppeliers & Broesterhuizen, 2007) contains references to other models in its glossary and an extensive bibliography.

More than 25 years later, SGT is still a new, exciting and controversial approach to working with psychosexual issues. This is one of its great attractions, but it won't, I believe, sell itself very easily, especially to other practitioners, without a context, both present and historical. This book will go some way towards filling the gaps identified above and will also present some ideas about the future direction of Willem Poppeliers' work.

The book will be divided into four main sections. The first will be devoted to an exploration of the ways in which psychosexual and relationship issues have been addressed from the deep past up to the present day, in the process of which the influences on the development of SGT will be highlighted. I've used the word 'addressed' here deliberately since I will not only be talking about the alleviation of psychosexual and relationship *problems* but also exploring how sex and relationships were thought about. The history of sex and relationships is clearly a huge subject, and it isn't my intention to explore it exhaustively. Foucault's *History of Sexuality* (Foucault, 1990a; 1990b; 1990c) ran to three volumes and was originally published over a period of approximately eight years and *A Cultural History of Sexuality* (Peakman, 2010) runs to six volumes! Whilst I can recommend both of these as useful background reading, what I want to do here is to outline a context or background within which Willem Poppeliers developed his ideas and that will enable the reader to connect with what they are reading. It's always easier to understand a new idea when you can hook it onto an idea that you may have already come across.

The second part of the book will locate SGT in the context of current thinking about sex and relationships and how issues with these are worked with professionally. The Western sexual revolution in the 1970s undoubtedly brought with it liberation from previous constraints and ultimately led to the considerable improvement, especially in the quantity and quality of the information available and the comparative tolerance (still not ideal by any means) that exists in the 21st century. However, the sexual nirvana that was imagined while these battles were being fought in the 20th century, from D. H. Lawrence (Lawrence, 2006) to Kinsey (Reinisch, 1991), Masters and Johnson (Masters & Johnson, 1988) and Hite (Hite, 1976) – not to mention Reich and the post-Reichians, has failed to materialise. Psychosexual and relationship issues remain as prevalent as ever. Again, I'm not aiming for an exhaustive survey here but rather an overview of current thinking and practice within the therapeutic, in its broadest sense, community. This means I will be looking not only at psychotherapeutic approaches to sexuality but also to what I refer to as 'non-mainstream' approaches such as Tantra and Sexological Bodywork.

The third part of the book will give a detailed description of the SGT model and its therapeutic application and organisation. In his developmental model, Willem Poppeliers addresses human beings' needs at each of the stages of their psychosexual development, particularly as far as parental responses are concerned. This section will explore the connection between these and many of the contemporary issues that we as a society are concerned with regarding sexuality and its expression in relationships. I will also include a short case vignette in order to clarify the sort of issues to which the model can be applied.

The fourth part of this book will be speculative. I don't have a crystal ball and can't accurately predict how this work will develop in the future. However, I think it will be useful to outline some ideas about the possible application and development of Willem Poppeliers' work in the future, especially as far as its contribution to the overall sexual and emotional health of humanity is concerned. This is crucial/vitally important as we struggle with the challenges of current social and political developments. In this section I will also explore the future context of SGT, especially its place in relation to the emerging trends in psychotherapy and sexual expression, together with an exploration of its relationship with the world of science and research.

Note

1 Since I wrote my thesis, Notburga Fischer (2018) has published her book, *Reifestufen der Sexuallen Leibe* (*The Developmental Levels of Sexual Love*), which refers extensively to Sexual Grounding; however, since my German is limited, I can't really comment on it here.

References

Duffell, N., & Poppeliers, W. (2006). 'Finding the right spoon – Searching for paradise in reality'. *Self and Society*, 34(1): 5–12.

Fischer, N. (2002). Sexual rootedness and the capacity for loving. In T. Itten & M. Fischer (Eds.), *Jack Lee Rosenberg: Celebrating a master psychotherapist, a festschrift in honour of his 70th birthday – 1 Jan. 2002* (pp. 110–118). St. Gallen: IBP Books.

Fischer, N. (2018). *Reifstufen der Sexuallen Leibe*. Köln: Innenwelt Verlag.

Foucault, M. (1990a). *The history of sexuality, vol 1*. New York: Vintage.

Foucault, M. (1990b). *The history of sexuality, vol 2*. New York: Vintage.

Foucault, M. (1990c). *The history of sexuality, vol 3*. New York: Vintage.

Hite, S. (1976). *A nationwide study of female sexuality*. New York: Collier MacMillan.

Lawrence, D. H. (2006). *Lady Chatterly's lover*. London: Wordsworth Classics.

Masters, W. H., & Johnson, V. E. (1988). *Sex and human loving*. New York: Little Brown.

Reinisch, J. M. (1991). *The Kinsey new report on sex*. London: St Martin's Press.

Peakman, J. (Ed.) (2010). *A cultural history of sexuality* (Vols. 1–6). Oxford: Bloomsbury.

Poppeliers, W., & Broesterhuizen, M. (2007). *Sexual grounding therapy*. Breda: Protocol Media Productions.

Part 1

Exploration

Chapter 1

History

There is no such thing as an original idea, model or theory if by 'original' we mean that the idea, model or theory has been produced in a vacuum. All ideas are either developments of existing ideas or reactions to them. Sometimes there are new, creative angles, which can unlock 'stuckness' and bring insight to bear on a problem, but these angles are almost always developed in the context of existing thought and knowledge. It is important for a newcomer to an idea, model or theory to be aware of the context in which it was developed in order to move from their familiar ground into new territory.

In this chapter, I am aiming to present a picture of the historical background against which Sexual Grounding Therapy (SGT) – its development, theory and practice – will be shown in sharp relief as the book unfolds.

As Ellenberger (1970) suggests in *The Discovery of the Unconscious*, the earliest ways of supporting healthy psychological development, which would have included sexuality and relationships, were connected with or part of religion. In prehistoric times, the way in which this help and support was given was part of the existing oral culture and cannot be directly accessed or researched. We are therefore dependent, as far as our understanding is concerned, on anthropological research (carried out by authors such as Malinowski and Mead in the early 20th century) into the way sex and relationships were lived and, where necessary, healed in the surviving indigenous cultures of that time. Wilhelm Reich (1971), one of Freud's followers and a pioneer of sexual liberation, drew on Malinowski's work in *The Invasion of Compulsory Sex-Morality*.

We also have the writings of indigenous authors such as Sobonfu Somé (1997) to give us a first-hand and more recent account. Without romanticising tribal cultures either in the past or in the present, we can see that one consequence of living in close contact and harmony with nature is that you are inevitably more at home with your own inner nature, including and especially your sexual nature. This means that the support that would almost certainly have been given to individuals with their psychosexual development would have been a matter of supporting that nature within the individual human being and within their social group. The flavour of this pervades Somé's *The Spirit of Intimacy* (1997). She talks movingly of the whole village community supporting the couple in negotiating the obstacles that inevitably arise during the course of an intimate relationship:

> In the Dagra community marriage is not a private matter. It's not just two individuals getting married. In fact, when a couple gets married, they create an occasion for other people to renew their vows and get married once again, at the same time. Sharing is a way of enlisting support for when problems start to hit.
>
> (p. 74)

I particularly appreciate the way that she assumes there *will* be problems and that support is available from the whole village to make the relationship the best it can be. The couple don't have to hide their problems behind closed doors and neither are they being sold a romantic myth. Of course, this system is dependent on a generational level of sex-positive and nature-positive support, which is rare in the 21st century and was under threat even as Somé was writing.

As the Abrahamic religions spread throughout the Middle East and Europe, it may not surprise us to observe that, although some support for psychological and psychosexual well-being might be offered within the context of the religious establishment, support for what would now be called healthy sexual expression became limited. In contrast to the 'tribal' approach, the Abrahamic approach is characterised by control and limitation (the oft quoted book of Leviticus being a prime example of this). In *Oedipus Revisited*, Shere Hite (2007), author of two groundbreaking surveys on male and female sexuality in the 20th century, suggests that some of the sexual prohibitions in Leviticus were in fact designed to increase the population of the Hebrew tribes, who had recently returned from exile, by limiting permissible sexual expression to 'foreplay followed by intercourse and ending with male orgasm inside the vagina' (Hite, 2007, p. 32).

Whether the kind of limitation and control I'm talking about is inevitable or necessary is an important question which will re-emerge throughout this book, but the fact that the context in which all three of these religions (Judaism, Christianity and Islam) developed was patriarchal almost certainly had something to do with it. Of course, I'm aware that patriarchy developed and still exists in other religious communities, but I'm focussing on the Abrahamic religions here, firstly because they are arguably dominant in the 21st century and secondly because patriarchy is enshrined within their monotheism.

At a very basic level in a patriarchal society, men, especially powerful men, are concerned to know that their sons are their sons, whereas women *always* know that their sons and daughters are their sons and daughters. Limiting the support given to what we in the 21st century might see as healthy sexual expression could be viewed as a way of preserving monogamy (and even polygamy, but definitely not polyandry!) and therefore reassuring the men concerned.

'Reassuring' is a very important word here, particularly where sex is concerned. Sexual desire sometimes seems irrational and has been argued by many, particularly poets and mystics, to be in itself, a form of madness. Where men and women are not supported in becoming self-regulating and self-fulfilled as they grow up, as they were in earlier cultures and which they unfortunately are not in the present day, then sex, along with death, becomes something to be feared. We could perhaps say that it is the life force, manifesting itself sexually and following its natural trajectory through maturation towards death, that is really what human beings have been afraid of since earliest times. In pagan cultures, this fear was contained and channelled (regulated, we might say in an SGT context) through ritual and licence, as, for example, in the Dionysian rites, where a degree of divine, sexual madness was supported. Pagan religions were also balanced, i.e., they had masculine *and* feminine principles enshrined within the pantheon of their divine beings, which gave a model for balancing the masculine and feminine parts of each human being; this balance is an essential ingredient of the self-regulation and self-fulfilment which I shall explore in Part 3 of this book.

With the coming of Christianity, or rather with its development as the state religion of the Roman Empire, the separation between the divine or rational aspects of human beings and their physical/emotional nature became even more extreme. Spirit and body came to be regarded as separate, the former being seen as superior to the latter and thinking being similarly privileged over feeling. Arguably, this separation between spirit and matter could be said to have started with the post-Socratic Greek philosophers, notably with Plato's doctrine of divine originals, but it became more pronounced as the Christian era developed. It was almost inevitable that, because the divine/rational seemed to offer more certainty in the face of the fear referred to in the previous paragraph, it should control and dominate the physical/emotional ever more strongly.

The contemporary writer and spiritual teacher Eckhart Tolle (1997), who quotes Jesus' teachings and parables in *The Power of Now*, clearly takes a different view of Christianity, seeing its essential message as *connecting* the divine with the physical rather than separating them, imbuing the body with spirit, rather than seeing the two as enemies; I am more in sympathy with this view. However, he makes it clear that he's talking about the essence of Christianity, Jesus as a spiritual teacher, rather than the institution of the church. Tolle draws on the teachings of Jesus (see Luke 12:27) in support of the idea that living in the here and now does away with the necessity of fear and control, and his recommended way of living in the present is through awareness of the body.

The control and domination that gradually developed as Christianity became an established institution were epitomised by the doctrine of original sin – that human beings, by their very nature and because of the fact that Eve, the first woman, had succumbed to the temptation of the serpent in the garden of Eden, are intrinsically sinful and need to be controlled from the outside, usually by a combination of the church and the state. It is possible, as Reich (1975) said in *The Mass Psychology of Fascism*, to see this as some kind of conspiracy where the control is being imposed on passive victims. The problem is that there's a circular process in operation here. The more we believe that part of us is sinful and needs controlling, the more we fear it and the more likely we are to believe that we need to be controlled from the outside. This can lead to us welcoming rather than resisting the externally imposed control. Reich (1945) described this situation as the 'emotional plague' (Reich, 1945, pp. 248–280) and used the idea to explain the rise of the far right in Germany and Austria in the 1920s and 1930s. Reich also believed that, by controlling the 'sinful' part of ourselves or having it controlled, the impulse we are afraid of will become more powerful and emerge in a destructive way, which supports the belief that it needed controlling in the first place.

Certainly, sexual experience and behaviour in the Middle Ages (as evidenced in Boccaccio's *The Decameron* and Chaucer's *The Canterbury Tales*), despite or maybe because of the draconian restrictions placed on sexual expression in that era, would support Reich's assertion. Put simply, there were a lot of rules and restrictions placed on the expression of sexuality. The fact that these were often ignored was used as evidence of their necessity in the first place.

The fear of sex and death (the fear of life?) is perhaps always a possibility for human beings who are 'blessed' with an enlarged neocortex, which enables us to learn, in a very sophisticated way, from past experience. We can project ourselves into the future and plan, but we can also generate within us a fear of that future and a seemingly insatiable desire for certainty. This makes us all very vulnerable to anyone, a priest, a politician or even a psychotherapist, who seems to be able to offer us that certainty in return for separating us even further from that part of us which makes us feel uncertain, i.e., our human (sexual) nature. Curiously, if we can accept this uncertainty both inside and outside ourselves and can learn to live with it in both senses of that word, our need for outside control diminishes. Our lives become exciting just by virtue of our being alive and then we don't have to look for external excitement in thrill-seeking activities.

It is important to note that the repression and control over its followers' sexuality, which gradually developed in the Christian establishment, was not universal. Within or just outside the 'system' there have always been individuals who recognise the unity of humanity and the importance of the life force in the whole of the cosmos. One such example was Hildegard von Bingen (1994). Hildegard was a visionary, musician and healer in 12th-century Germany and, although she had some peculiar ideas about the physiology of conception and birth (that the man plants his seed in the woman, whose role is then to nurture that seed with her menstrual blood in order for the seed to mature into a human being), she at least acknowledges sexual desire and pleasure in both sexes. In stating that healthy women maintain that desire into their seventies, she also acknowledges that there is more to sex between men and women than reproduction, which is what the church was teaching.

This position of being on the fringes of the mainstream is also, as will be explored in the fourth part of this book, where I believe psychotherapy and especially SGT, truly belongs. Arthur Versluis (2008), in *The Secret History of Western Sexual Mysticism*, takes a similar but different position on the relationship between religion and sexuality, thinking more in terms of the pagan/early Christian sexual rituals described earlier being preserved and perpetuated in secret and underground rather than visibly on the fringes. These included the Dionysian rites and, most importantly, other rituals designed to allow worshipers to experience the relationship between the divine masculine and the divine feminine, which according to Versluis, have been preserved from the pre-Christian era and incorporated into the beliefs of some Christian sects until the present day.

Help for emotional, relationship and sexual problems continued to be available through the church during the Renaissance mostly, as Ellenberger documents, via the casting out of 'demons' along with the kind of pastoral support that, however kindly meant it might have been in individual cases, essentially reinforced the restrictive status quo. The recognition of human beings as entities in their own right as a byproduct of the Enlightenment seemed like a significant step forward. However, McGilchrist (2009) argues that the Enlightenment, by prizing left brain over right, separated human beings even further from their own nature by prizing rationality rather than a judgemental divine being. I would suggest that the post-Socratic Greek philosophers began this process earlier by linking the rational with the divine, but, interestingly, Freud, who was known to be a classical scholar before he undertook his medical training, shows the considerable influence of this way of thinking in the development of psychoanalysis. Clearly the philosophy of the Enlightenment gives human beings more sense of autonomy, but the price of this is separation from themselves, which I shall discuss further in Chapter 3.

The overall support for individual human beings expressing their sexuality and life energy as human beings was to remain limited until towards the end of the 19th century when the first sexologists, Havelock Ellis and Richard Kraft-Ebbing, began to write about sexuality. Notwithstanding their focus on the pathological aspects of sexuality, these two authors amongst others represent the beginning of a movement to study sexuality as a serious scientific subject and a 'respectable' branch of medicine. It is significant that neither of these pioneers were ordinary members of respectable society and that they both opened themselves up to considerable criticism and censure for bringing sexuality into the public arena.

In parallel with this development, Jean-Martin Charcot, a respected and pioneering neurologist, was using hypnotism to cure his patients at the Salpêtrière hospital in Paris. Hypnotism, as Ellenberger (1970) observes, had been used to alleviate emotional distress since the 18th century when Anton Mesmer, a Viennese physician and hypnotist, was reputed to have cast doubt on the efficacy of the work of the exorcist, Gastner, at a commission of enquiry. Mesmer's success in duplicating the processes, which had previously been attributed to exorcism, according to Ellenberger, marked the end of the dominance of the church over the population's emotional well-being (Ellenberger, 1970, pp. 56–57).

Charcot made some important contributions to the field of psychosexual therapy. Previously, hysteria had been thought only to affect women, an idea which dates back to ancient Egyptian times when it was thought to be caused by the womb (*hystera* in Greek) becoming displaced and wandering around the body. Charcot began to see that the condition, which was sometimes characterised by symptoms such as unexplained paralysis or inability to speak and sometimes by 'extreme' sexual behaviour, was psychological in origin and could affect both men and women (Goetz, 1987) (This idea was to become very important in the work of W. H. R. Rivers with trauma victims during the first world war, although the word 'hysteric' was never used to describe victims of shell shock, who were said to be suffering from neurasthenia). However, most of Charcot's patients *were* women and, although there was little doubt that he used them, some would say shamelessly, to increase his own prestige in the medical world, he also brought relief to many patients who may otherwise have simply been incarcerated in asylums.

Charcot also believed that sexual dysfunction was an underlying cause of hysteria, famously stating in a discussion with a colleague and within Freud's hearing: 'Mais, dans des cas pareils, c'est toujours la chose génitale, toujours! toujours! toujours!' ['But, in cases like this, it's always something sexual, always! always! always!'] (Reich, 1973, p. 95).

Freud was later to write in his diary: 'I know that for a moment I was paralysed with astonishment and I said to myself "Yes, but if he knows this, why does he never say so?"' (Reich, 1973 p. 95).

I recently came across a possible answer to this question of Freud's, which Reich was later to ask of Freud himself. Doctors had, since the time of Hippocrates, been routinely giving genital massage, either themselves or via midwives, to their female patients in order to 'cure' their hysteria. However, this was neither considered a sexual act, because it didn't involve penetration by a man, nor was it greatly talked or written about other than in learned journals. This practice was researched by Rachel Maines (1999) in *The Technology of Orgasm* where she asserts that the vibrator was developed by doctors to relieve them of the manual effort involved! The answer, then, is in another example of the kind of double standard which patriarchal society applies to female sexuality. The statement made by male doctors seems to be something like, 'We will acknowledge, in private and in our learned writings, the importance and existence of female sexual desire, but, to preserve our reputations, we will treat it as a symptom or pathology which needs to be cured and we won't speak about it publicly'.

It is significant that Freud and Breuer were surprised (Breuer was 'traumatised'!) that 'Dora', their first patient, developed an intense erotic transference towards Breuer when he was routinely giving her warm baths and massages alongside her psychological treatment (Freud & Breuer, 1991).

Freud was clearly a pioneer in bringing the connection between neurosis in both men and women and sexual dysfunction into the open along with the idea of psychosexual development, the Oedipus complex and infantile sexuality generally. Like most pioneers, especially social pioneers, Freud put a lot of his energy into getting his ideas accepted by the (medical) establishment of his time. In *Freud and his Followers*, Paul Roazen (1992) details the restrictions on Freud, as a Jew, being accepted by the Austrian establishment in any field and how, even though medicine was one profession where Jews *were* accepted, Freud himself was open about his wish for psychoanalysis not just to be known as a Jewish profession and organisation, hence his enthusiasm for Jung being involved. When we look at it from a 21st-century perspective, this difficulty with being accepted can be seen to have skewed his work and the way it developed during his lifetime. Freud was also a man, and I use that word advisedly, of his time and this can be seen to have influenced his ideas on sexuality in general and women's sexuality in particular. I will make further reference to this influence in Chapter 3.

So, when Freud first began to develop the theory of psychoanalysis, he emphasised the idea of 'libido' or sexual/life energy, how it could be repressed and how that repression could be moderated in order that his patients could live more fulfilled lives. As the theory and organisation of psychoanalysis developed, it seemed to become more of a method of maintaining the status quo than the liberating force that seemed possible in its early days (Freud, 2010). The 'superego' became more prominent as a restraining force on the chaotic 'id' and the theory of the 'death instinct' was arguably partly developed as a way of explaining patients' resistance and seems to constitute a version of the Christian idea of original sin.

In creating this other, negative drive, psychoanalysis, especially in the work of Melanie Klein (1984), endorses the idea of a part of us that is intrinsically negative and potentially out of control and another part that is responsible for doing the controlling. Practised from this perspective, psychoanalysis potentially separates human beings from their own nature. This is not so much in the emphasis being on making the unconscious conscious but in the subsuming of the now conscious impulses of a chaotic id into the service of the mature 'ego', the superego being the agent of control. Again, this control and separation is designed to counter our fear of the life, both inside all of us individually and, regrettably, in society as a whole, as Freud (2010) explored in *Civilisation and its Discontents*. However, like most defensive strategies whose aim is to counter or reduce fear, whether individual or societal, this one only increases it.

It was left to Reich (1973; Sharaf, 1983) to re-invigorate psychoanalysis, both by bringing back the idea that a free flow of libido was a sign of psychophysical health and also by re-radicalising the work. Reich brought the connection between sexual dysfunction and neurosis back into the psychoanalytic movement and developed methods that worked with resistance, which the older psychoanalysts had previously seen as a problem to be overcome before the analysis could really begin. He also brought the body and its energy into the work, thus reversing the trend of separation between mind and body that began centuries before and was epitomised by Descartes' dualism.

Reich was also aware of and worked with the social applications of psycho-analytic ideas in a way that the early psychoanalytic movement, under Freud and his successors disapproved of and did not use. In cooperation with fellow Marxists, he gave public lectures and advice sessions to young people about sexual health and worked in psychoanalytic polyclinics, which were centres where poor people could obtain psychoanalytic treatment at little or no cost.

If Freud was a man of his time, then Reich was even more so. Working in the ideological ferment of post-World War I Austria, he had little incentive to be accepted by the political and social establishment, although his later obsession with being accepted by the scientific community was to consume a large amount of his energy and efforts and, arguably, led to his downfall. He was therefore able to focus his work on sex and the physicality of sex, together with its relationship with neurosis. He recognised the relationship between fear and control, which I referred to earlier as 'the emotional plague', not only in individual human beings but also in society, and he was able to remain sufficiently outside the establish-ment, including the psychoanalytic establishment, for his ideas not to have become distorted into support for the *status quo*.

Staying on the outside of the establishment, at least for the first part of his life, enabled Reich to encourage and support the natural sexual impulses of his patients and to advocate this support in fellow practitioners. These included not only his fellow analysts but also others to whose work such ideas had relevance, notably A. S. Neill, a prominent and also controversial educationalist in the early 20th cen-tury. As Reich's career developed, his intense desire to have his ideas accepted by the (medical/scientific) establishment, together with his disappointment at being essentially rejected by the political left, seemed to lead to a withdrawal from his focus on personal and social sexual liberation. It was as if the illusory scientific acceptance would somehow compensate for the lack of societal acceptance of his founding ideas about human energy and sexuality, especially, as he had hoped, in America. It is interesting to note that both Freud and Reich were disappointed by the reception of their work in America, although a version of Freud's work, with which he was less than happy, did catch on there (It became highly medicalised and the concept of 'cure' was established).

In his dealings with the world thereafter, Reich seems to have taken refuge in his identity as a pioneering scientist, which culminated in his refusal to accept that the American courts had the capacity to judge his ideas about orgone energy, since none of them were fellow scientists. It was therefore left to his followers to bring his revolutionary therapeutic work to the world, each of whom did this in their own way (Sharaf, 1983).

One of the most prominent amongst Reich's successors was Alexander Lowen who, whilst building on Reich's work with sexual energy and intro-ducing some important innovations such as working with clients standing up and getting them to feel the contact they were making with the ground ('grounding'), seems to have taken the work in a more mainstream direction, reminiscent of the 'American dream' of the 1950s and 1960s. It cannot be denied that, in the latter years of his disappointment with his lack of acceptance by the scientific community and by the therapy establishment in America, Reich became more and more extreme in his theories and less and less focused on clinical work. Something needed to change and his successors, of whom Lowen was one, refocused his work in a more realistic and clinical direction.

Perhaps as a response to the social climate – this was, after all, the McCarthy era – as much as to the more eccentric of Reich's ideas about flying saucers and weather control, Lowen brought the concept of 'cure' into the work, as had the American analysts, along with certainty and control. His work therefore became more recognised by the therapeutic and medical establishment and gained Lowen a large following in Europe and in the Americas. My own experience of bioenergetic therapy between the mid 1970s and early 1980s was that there was certainly an acknowledgement of the importance of sex and the sexual nature of bodily energy, the goal of the work being to unblock the flow of energy in order to become a fulfilled human being. There was also an emphasis on putting the body under stress so that 'giving in' to the flow of energy was almost inevitable. There was, it seemed to me, an equal emphasis on money and success as signs that we were moving our energy appropriately in the world. Although Willem Poppeliers wouldn't necessarily embrace all of these ideas, Lowen's Bioenergetics had a profound effect on the development of the Sexual Grounding model, which I shall write about in the next chapter.

To summarise: this chapter has presented a brief account of how human beings have been helped with their sexual problems, whether the emphasis has been on curing the problems or on promoting sexual fulfilment. This has involved some exploration of the different ways human beings have thought about sex and about their own nature. What emerges from this exploration is the tension between sexual (life) impulses and control, particularly the perceived necessity of external control. This will become a theme in this book.

References

Boccacio, G. (2003). *The decameron* (G. H. McWilliam, Trans.). London: Penguin.

Chaucer, G. (2003). *The Canterbury tales* (N. Coghill, Trans.). London: Penguin.

Ellenberger, H. F. (1970). *The discovery of the unconscious*. New York: Harper Collins.

Freud, S., & Breuer, J. (1991). *Studies in hysteria*. London: Penguin.

Freud, S. (2010). *Civilisation and its discontents*. New York: W.W. Norton & Co.

Goetz, C. G. (1987). *Charcot, the clinician*. New York: Raven Press.

Hite, S. (2007). *Oedipus revisited*. London: Arcadia Books Ltd.

Klein, M. (1984). *Envy and gratitude and other works, 1946–1963*. London: The Hogarth Press.

McGilchrist, I. (2009). *The master and his emissary*. London: Yale University Press.

Maines, R. P. (1999). *The technology of orgasm*. Baltimore, MD: Johns Hopkins University Press.

New English Bible. (1961). Oxford: Oxford University Press.

Reich, W. (1945). *Character analysis*. New York: Noonday Press.

Reich, W. (1971). *The invasion of compulsory sex-morality*. London: Pelican.

Reich, W. (1973). *The function of the orgasm*. New York: Noonday Press.

Reich, W. (1975). *The mass psychology of fascism*. London: Pelican.

Roazen, P. (1992). *Freud and his followers*. New York: Da Capo Press.

Sharaf, M. (1983). *Fury on earth*. New York: Da Capo Press.

Somé, S. (1997). *The spirit of intimacy*. New York: William Morrow.

Tolle, E. (1997). *The power of now*. Vancouver: Namaste Publishing.

Versluis, A. (2008). *The secret history of western sexual mysticism*. Rochester, VT: Inner Traditions International.

von Bingen, H. (1994). *Holistic healing*. Collegeville, MN: The Liturgical Press.

Chapter 2

Willem Poppeliers – his influences and the origins of Sexual Grounding Therapy

This chapter is based on an interview with Willem Poppeliers on 31 January, 2018 and on various follow-up conversations and email exchanges. It will trace the origins of, and influences on, Poppeliers' development of Sexual Grounding Therapy (SGT).

Poppeliers studied both developmental and clinical psychology at university. The training included psychoanalysis, Rogerian therapy and behavioural therapy and students were required to experience all three of these as clients/patients. After graduating, he underwent psychoanalysis and bioenergetic analysis and also experienced intensive Vegetotherapy (two blocks of 14 days with one session per day) as part of a project at Oslo University.

Poppeliers went on to train in bioenergetic analysis with Alexander Lowen as part of an international training in Belgium. After that, he began travelling and met with John Periakos in America and undertook short professional development courses with him. During his time in America, Poppeliers met Jack Painter and undertook training in the bodywork methods Painter had developed in the 1960s and early 1970s, Postural Integration and Energetic Integration. They became friends and colleagues, collaborating on an ambitious book project together as well as running international workshops and developing a body psychotherapy, which had the provisional name of 'Breath and Life'.

Poppeliers had been drawn to Lowen's work, as well as to the pioneering work of Reich. He and Painter had both felt that these ways of working with bodily energy, even though they acknowledged the sexual nature of the life energy they worked with, left the genitals out of the clinical work. It's true, of course, that Reich, in the scientific work he carried out in Europe before the World War II, researched genital excitement and orgasm in both men and women and his work on orgastic potency revolutionised the perception of men's, and by implication women's, sexual problems. Up until this point, a man was presumed to be sexually healthy if he could achieve an erection and ejaculate (preferably inside a woman). Reich, on the other hand, defined sexual health, or orgastic potency, as 'the capacity to surrender to the flow of biological energy, free from any inhibitions; the capacity to discharge completely the dammed-up sexual excitation through involuntary, pleasurable convulsions of the body'

(Reich, 1973, p. 102). This meant that a large number of men who had previously been thought by the psychoanalytic establishment to be sexually healthy but whose neuroses had non-sexual origins were in fact suffering from profound sexual disturbance. In this way, Reich refuted the challenge to his idea, taken originally from Freud's early work, that *all* neurosis had a sexual aetiology (see the Charcot anecdote quoted in the previous chapter).

Willem Poppeliers had observed that there were two things missing from the body-centred approaches he was encountering in Europe and America. The first was the absence of working directly with the genitals themselves as relational parts of the body in a clinical setting, even though individuals would certainly have energetic blocks in this area. This was and is controversial, mostly because of the way it might be perceived by the general public and by the psychotherapeutic establishment, but also because of the difficulties it presents in terms of the transference and counter-transference in the therapy relationship. I will comment further on this later in this chapter and more extensively in Part 3 of this book. Poppeliers had become aware that, although they had involved the pelvis in their early therapeutic work, bioenergetic therapists, including Lowen himself, were focusing on it less and less as the model developed and became more established.

The second thing that Poppeliers brought to the field of bodywork was the idea of working with the client relationally, that is to say being aware of and working within the transference and counter-transference and also viewing the client as a relational being. In his early work, Reich worked a lot with transference and counter-transference, one of his contributions being to advocate the encouragement and exploration of negative transference (see Reich, 1945). Once he began to bring the body more explicitly into the therapeutic process, he became more interested in the flow of energy within the individual body rather than the exchange of energy between human beings in relationship. In bringing the relationship into bodywork, Willem Poppeliers was incorporating the influence of the object relations school of psychoanalysis, the emphasis being on the relationship within which the energy is expressed rather than the flow or expression itself.

One of the key concepts in object relations is that of maternal mirroring (Winnicott, 1967; 1986). Babies, at an early stage of development, need to have themselves reflected back by their mothers in order to confirm their existence. This is the fundamental basis of a healthy secure relationship – 'I have the right to be me relating to you and experiencing myself as a subject relating to an object.' Otherwise, where the child hasn't received good enough mirroring, usually because the parent is demanding to be mirrored by the child rather than the other way round, the child will go on to form relationships based on the latter experience. They will develop what Winnicott calls a 'false self' based on the child's anticipation of what the parent wants. In this, the statement to him/herself is, 'I can be me as long as I give mummy or daddy the response they want'.

In developing the Sexual Grounding model, Poppeliers incorporated the concept of mirroring into the dynamic between parents and children at the Oedipal stage of development, where what is being mirrored is the child as a sexual being rather than their existence. This is consistent with Lowen's theory of character structure, which was influential on Poppeliers in the development of the Sexual Grounding model. Character structure has sometimes been expressed as a series of 'rights'. With the schizoid character structure (Lowen, 1959), which belongs to an age which is the focus of Winnicott's object relations theory described above, what is at issue is the right to exist. However, with the Oedipal character structures, the phallic narcissistic and hysterical, it's the right to be a sexual being.

Having begun to work with Jack Painter as a colleague (the process of moving from being a trainee to being a colleague seems to have evolved organically), Poppeliers began to link his ideas around bringing sexuality and relationship into body psychotherapy with the Postural Integration and Energetic Integration which Painter had himself developed. Bringing the sexuality/sexual energy and relationship into the bodywork in these early days involved a lot of hands on work on the part of the therapist, whether this was in an individual or a group setting.

From the start, Poppeliers was keen to have a tight ethical code in place for this work in order that clients would feel safe and also to enable the work to be more widely accepted in the world. More than that, if the work was relational, it meant that transference and counter-transference would be part of that relationship, which in turn meant that both therapists and clients needed to feel safe to explore these aspects of the therapeutic relationship safely and professionally.

Painter, on the other hand, seems to have believed that clients in therapy were autonomous adults who were capable of making their own decisions about their therapeutic boundaries, including whether or not they chose to have sex with their therapist. When Poppeliers challenged him on this, Painter's counter-argument seems to have been that Poppeliers, like a lot of psychodynamic psychotherapists and especially analysts, didn't want to let his clients grow up.

In making sense of this, it has to be remembered that, as far as I can tell from reading his obituary, whilst Painter 'personally explored' many different kinds of humanistic and body psychotherapies, his background was in philosophy and psychology but doesn't seem to have included formal psychotherapy training. Indeed, he insisted that Postural Integration, Energetic Integration and Pelvic-Heart Integration were *not* psychotherapies but forms of personal exploration and growth (Zeihl, 2010).

A lot of Painter's 'personal' exploration was in the 1960s and 1970s, a period in which there was a lot of revolt against the rigidity of the psychoanalytic establishment. This revolt was especially against the aspects of power and control which were definitely seen to be, and in many cases were, implicit in its culture. It isn't surprising, therefore, that he might not have wanted to recognise the existence and power of the transference relationship in his work and he was certainly not alone in this. Jeffrey Masson famously alludes to the use/abuse of transference and counter-transference to support his critique of the entire therapy profession (Masson, 1988).

As someone whose involvement with personal growth goes back to the 1970s, I can say that this attitude, certainly as far as power, transference, mainstream psychotherapy etc., were concerned, was not uncommon in that era. My route into therapy was via the Diploma in Applied Behavioural Sciences course based at what was then North London Polytechnic (now the University of North London). The work there was as political/social as it was psychotherapeutic and, although the course leader, John Southgate, was a follower of Reich both politically and therapeutically and went on to found the Centre for Attachment Based Psychotherapy, many of the students and staff would probably have agreed with Jack Painter's rejection of analytic rules and regulations, as we might have seen them.

Most of the therapies/growth work I was involved with in the early 1970s didn't specifically focus on sexuality or involve hands-on work. Bioenergetics, with which I became involved in 1975, clearly did involve hands-on contact between therapist and client but had very strict boundaries around touch. When I first started bioenergetic therapy as a client, we worked in underwear, but it's interesting to note that this gradually changed during the time I was involved in the work, with women beginning to wear leotards and men to wear tracksuits or shorts. Rumour had it that there was a bioenergetic therapist somewhere in the UK who did work with his clients naked, but this was definitely frowned upon in the training group of which I became a part in the early 1980s.

Poppeliers' response, at the time, to Painter's accusation that he didn't want to let his clients grow up centred more on Poppeliers' wish to operate in the same manner as the health professions, which he believed kept both practitioner and patient safe. This makes a lot of sense, but I have a different though not mutually exclusive way of looking at it. Compared to many forms of (particularly psychodynamic) psychotherapy, SGT is unique in that it *insists* that clients do grow up, particularly as it focuses on adult stages of psychosexual development as the model unfolds. However, whilst doing this, SGT also focuses on the function of parents throughout clients' lives, up to and including death (see Part 3). In this sense, the transference and counter-transference remains an issue throughout the client's involvement with SGT.

In writing this book, I have had contact with practitioners who, after the split between Painter and Poppeliers, continued to practise Postural Integration, Energetic Integration and Painter's equivalent of SGT, Pelvic-Heart Integration (PHI) (I learned quite a lot about PHI from a useful Skype conversation with Dirk Marivoet, who is the General Secretary of the International Council of PsychoCoporal Integration Trainers, and I will discuss this more fully in Chapter 4). What became clear from these conversations was that there was clearly some cross fertilisation between what each of these two men brought to the work they did together. Separating exactly who contributed what is beyond the scope of this book, but it was clearly a painful separation for both parties and also for those who were close to them at the time. In my interview with him, Poppeliers was clear that, after the separation with Painter, he took all of Painter's work out of the Sexual Grounding model. From my brief overview, however, there is a lot in the PHI model that is very familiar to a Sexual Grounding Trainer.

One thing that is widely known about Poppeliers is that he is a prolific thinker, writer and visionary. The impression I have developed during my involvement with SGT over 12 years, and which has since been confirmed in one of my many conversations with Poppeliers himself, is that there was a lot of material, in terms of structures, exercises etc. that he developed around this time. For organisational reasons, the trainings that Poppeliers began to offer in the 1990s under the auspices of Bodymind, a body psychotherapy training institute based in Holland, and that came to form what we at first called the Basic and Advanced courses (now called Coursework 1 & 2) in SGT had to be shortened and a lot of Poppeliers' original structures and exercises had to be left out. It may be that these could be developed by the organisation in the future and offered as a follow-up to the coursework (see Part 4).

The original trainings Willem Poppeliers offered with Jack Painter seem to be what we would now call Continuing Professional Development and were aimed at professional practitioners whose work involved sexuality. I will be referring to this possible direction for the SGT work in Part 4 of this book. After the separation, Poppeliers developed and began to offer Coursework 1 and 2 as therapy/personal growth, in the way I shall describe in Part 3, first with Bodymind in Holland and later in Mexico and internationally.

More recently, Poppeliers has scaled down his involvement with the clinical side of SGT and no longer facilitates workshops himself. He is now more interested in promoting links with the scientific community and I will explore this further in Chapter 17.

In this chapter I have outlined Willem Poppeliers' development as a practitioner and the influences on his work from the early days of his training up to the time when he developed the model that became Coursework 1 and 2 as they are practised today.

References

Lowen, A. (1959). *The language of the body*. New York: Collier Books.
Masson, J. (1988). *Against therapy*. Monroe, ME: Common Courage Press.
Reich, W. (1945). *Character analysis*. New York: Noonday Press.
Reich, W. (1973). *The function of the orgasm*. New York: Noonday Press.
Winnicott, D. W. (1967). Mirror-role of the mother and family in child development. In P. Lomas (Ed.), *The predicament of the family: A psycho-analytical symposium* (pp. 26–33). London: Hogarth.

Winnicott, D. W. (1986). *Home is where we start from*. London: Pelican.
Zeihl, S. (2010). 'Obituary for Jack Painter'. Gent: International Community of Psychocorporal (Bodymind) Integration Trainers and Practitioners. Available at: www.icpit.org/jack-w-painter

Part 2

Comparison

Introduction to Part 2

In the UK at the moment, there are more psychotherapists and counsellors than there ever have been, probably in absolute terms and almost certainly per head of the population. According to the British Association for Counselling and Psychotherapy (BACP) website, there are 96 accredited training courses in counselling (BACP, 2021) and, according to the United Kingdom Council for Psychotherapy (UKCP) website, 'around 80 organisations who offer training or accreditation to allow psychotherapists to become a member of UKCP' (UKCP, 2020). Even if each course only graduates 10 students (and this is a very conservative estimate) this means that nearly 2,000 practitioners are entering the profession every year.

If this army of psychotherapists and counsellors were effectively addressing the UK's sexual problems, we would be a much healthier nation, in terms of our sexuality, but recent research suggests otherwise (Mitchell et al., 2013). Divorce and relationship breakdown statistics, not to mention the prevalence of rape, sexual abuse and porn addiction, also present a worrying picture of the nation's sexual health. There is more information available about sex and relationships than in previous generations and these are frequently discussed in the press and social media, yet somehow the difficulties we experience around sexuality and relationships persist and increase.

It is also important to recognise that there are other ways of working with sexuality than through psychotherapy and counselling, especially when we see this work as developing/restoring the possibility of sexual fulfilment and not just about solving sexual 'problems'. These include Tantra, sex coaching, somatic coaching, somatic sexology, etc.

In this section I want to talk about some of the different models of working with sexuality and about how Sexual Grounding Therapy complements or is similar to these models and about how it differs, goes beyond them or even has something to learn from them. As I said in my introduction, I'm not going to attempt an exhaustive survey here. This would certainly be an interesting project for someone in the future to pick up, but my intention, having located Sexual Grounding Therapy historically in the last section, is to locate it in the present and to see where it fits in with other contemporary approaches and where it is perhaps in conflict.

References

British Association for Counselling and Psychotherapy (BACP). (2021). *Courses*. Lutterworth: British Assocation for Counselling and Psychotherapy. Available at: https://www.bacp.co.uk/search/Courses

Mitchell, K. R., Mercer, C. H., Ploubidis, G. B., Jones, K. G., Datta, J., Field, N., Copas, A. J., Tanton, C., Erens, B., Sonnenberg, P., Clifton, S., Macdowall, W., Phelps, A., Johnson, A. M., & Wellings, K. (2013). 'Sexual function in Britain: findings from the third National Survey of Sexual Attitudes and Lifestyles (Natsal-3)'. *Lancet*, 382, 1817–1829.

United Kingdom Council for Psychotherapy (UKCP). (2020). *Psychotherapy training*. London: UK Council for Psychotherapy. Available at: https://www.psychotherapy.org.uk/psychotherapy-training/

Chapter 3

Mainstream psychotherapy and counselling

Training

As part of the research for this book, I carried out an online survey using the tool SurveyMonkey, which allows users to carry out fairly spontaneous online enquiries into specific topics and to target potential respondents. There were two parts to this survey: the first was addressed to qualified counsellors and psychotherapists and the second to training providers. I used the Facebook Groups 'Counsellors Connect' and 'Counselling Private Practice' as my source for the first and the British Association for Counselling and Psychotherapy (BACP) list of accredited counselling courses for the second. I was asking about the quantity and quality of training input on psychosexual issues. By 'psychosexual issues' I was referring to any issues related to sex that a client might bring to counselling/psychotherapy. This could include problems in their sexual relationship, problems of sexual identity, shame and guilt about sexual feelings, fantasies and behaviour, etc.

My first significant finding was that, whilst I received over 80 responses from qualified practitioners, only 3 of the 80 or so training providers I contacted chose to respond. I could have pursued them for a response, but after some thought, I decided to leave the data as it was and to draw my own conclusions. It could be, of course, that training providers are overloaded with work, especially given the amount of paperwork involved in any kind of training these days, but I suspect that training providers were reluctant to reveal how little time they devoted to psychosexual issues in their training programmes.

Amongst the qualified practitioners, around 65% received one session or less of input on psychosexual issues. Around 54% received either unsatisfactory input or input focussed on symptoms/treatment. Over 73% either had no briefing at all on psychosexual issues in their placement or were encouraged to refer any clients who presented with psychosexual issues for sex therapy. Only 15% were encouraged to view erotic transference or counter-transference as possible growth points in the therapeutic relationship. For the rest, erotic transference/counter-transference was seen as a problem, viewed in terms of ethics and boundaries or not mentioned at all.

Surprisingly, nearly 70% of respondents said they felt 'completely comfortable' or 'fairly comfortable' working with psychosexual issues. I think I should have been more specific in my question here. Respondents who chose the 'other' option to this question (SurveyMonkey allows an 'other' option in the multiple-choice responses, which enables respondents to comment in their own words if they feel none of the choices offered expresses their view) made a distinction between 'comfortable' and 'competent'. I could possibly have rephrased the question to elicit responses that referred to the depth to which the psychosexual issues were being explored and the amount of initiative taken by the therapist.

As I expected, the overall indication is that most practitioners don't feel that they've had enough input on psychosexual issues in their training to be able to work with them effectively. Looking at the situation from a course provider's perspective, I might argue that time is limited on training courses, that psycho-sexual issues are a specialism and that, if students want to work with it, they have the option to undertake further training as part of the Continuing Professional Development (CPD) requirement of their accreditation/registration. There is truth in all of these statements, but we also have to look at the orientation, or psychotherapeutic model, of each mainstream training.

I will discuss different specific psychotherapeutic models later in this chapter. For now, it is important to note that, if the overall course model is relational and, as the two training courses I have been responsible for were, influenced by sex-positive practitioners, then it's more likely that sexuality and relationships will run through the training, like a central thread. Too often it is relegated, as some respondents remarked, to a one-off lecture sometimes delivered by an outside specialist. I remember that one of the essay titles I set my students when I was course leader at East Surrey College was 'Counselling which does not involve both the client's and the counsellor's sexual energy does not get to the heart of the matter. Discuss with reference to the work of Wilhelm Reich'.

My experience as an external examiner, together with anecdotal evidence from various practitioners I have come across in supervision and CPD courses I have run, leads me to believe that psychosexual issues are not fully addressed in most psychotherapy and counselling training. This means that the way a client's psychosexual issues, which arguably, if we are to believe Freud's original for-mulation and Reich's continuation of it, underpin most of the other issues that may be distressing them, are addressed in their therapy is dependent on the personal commitment and experience of the practitioner they choose to work with. Often, clients themselves aren't aware of the significance of these issues and therefore wouldn't necessarily look for a practitioner who overtly stated that they worked with them in their public profile.

A simple answer to the problem I'm raising here would be for BACP/ UKCP to revise their criteria for accredited courses, assuming they agreed with my view. Apart from being based on a questionable assumption, such a solution would raise two other issues. The first would be finding the staff who could teach this revised curriculum at depth. As I said earlier in this section, being a practitioner in a sex-positive model would be an important qualification, but, as will become apparent in the next part of this chapter, such models are rare in counselling and psychotherapy. The other issue would be that of deciding what these revised criteria would be.

My own experience in delivering the psychosexual component of the only course I've taught that I didn't at least have a hand in designing myself was that the focus was exclusively on 'problems' or, as I referred to it in my survey, 'symptoms/treatment'. This is understandable and may be consistent with some therapeutic models, but it's hardly sex-positive. Arriving at a universal definition of sexual (emotional) health may be a daunting task, but one thing it's not is an absence of symptoms. The World Health Organisation defined sexual health in 2006 as 'a state of physical, emotional, mental and social wellbeing in relation to sexuality; it is not merely an absence of disease, dysfunction or infirmity' (WHO, 2006). Another possible answer to the problem I pose in this section is that of raising awareness of the importance of psychosexual issues in everyday life, as pioneers like Freud and Reich intended, and feeding this through into mainstream trainings. This could be done via the 'applied SGT' which I discuss in Chapter 15 of this book.

Models of mainstream psychotherapy and counselling

It can sometimes seem as if there are almost as many different models of psychotherapy as there are practitioners working with them, and new models are evolving as I'm writing this book. However, for simplicity's sake I'm going to talk about three main streams of psychotherapy: the psychodynamic stream, which has its origins in the work of Sigmund Freud; the humanistic stream, which developed in the 1940s and 1950s with the work of Carl Rogers, Abraham Maslow, Irvin Yalom, etc.; and the behavioural/cognitive behavioural stream, originally developed by J. D. Watson and B. F. Skinner in the early 20th century and modified later by Aaron Beck and Albert Ellis.

These 'streams' are broad – rivers almost – and there is clearly much variation within each, with many practitioners and theorists crossing the streams and including elements of all three, arguably, in their models and, almost certainly, in the way they practise them. John Rowan (2005), in *The Future of Training in Psychotherapy and Counselling*, observes that, whilst it is relatively easy to distinguish newly qualified practitioners from each other according to the model that formed the basis of their training, it becomes much more difficult the more years of post-qualification experience they acquire. For the purpose of clarity, I will be treating them as discrete models.

Of the three streams I've mentioned, the psychodynamic stream is the one which most explicitly refers to sexuality and psychosexual issues. As I've said elsewhere (Lamb, 2017) and also in Chapter 1 of this book, Freud's pioneering work was important in that it put sexuality, and in particular childhood sexuality, firmly on the table in looking at our development as human beings. It also acknowledged unconscious process, particularly transference and counter-transference, and the importance of unconscious communication. I have also already referred to the concept of mirroring, which is an important part of the work of D. W. Winnicott and is also important in Sexual Grounding Therapy (SGT).

However, psychodynamic thought is fairly diverse and there are a considerable number of psychodynamic writers and practitioners who espouse a very different view of human sexuality to that which SGT offers. There is a determinism in the theories of some psychoanalytic writers, starting with Freud himself and including Jacques Lacan and Melanie Klein, that goes beyond Freud's concept of 'psychic determinism' (the idea that decisions and actions are mostly based on unconscious process rather than on rational thought) (Freud, 1969).

Lacan is perhaps one of the more extreme psychoanalytic thinkers of the mid-20th century; he saw it as his mission to return psychotherapy to the purity of Freud's original thoughts and concepts. Although not all psychoanalytic thinkers and practitioners are this extreme, I am using him as an example because he represents a strong current within the psychoanalytic stream of what could be seen as pessimism about the human condition.

To say that the interpretation of Lacan is problematic is an understatement. He makes no secret of the fact that he expresses his ideas in a way that is deliberately obscure – a conscious challenge to the reader to think! Part of me admires this, but it does make it difficult, even for readers with a sophisticated knowledge of psychotherapeutic theory, to understand. One result of *my* thinking, based on Roger Horrocks' account in his book on the study of sexuality, is that Lacan seems to be saying that all human desire is based on unfulfillable lack or loss – perhaps of the mother's breast or, in women, of a penis (Horrocks, 1997). I love the philosopher Hélène Cixous' robust and passionate response to this idea:

> I don't want a penis to decorate my body with. But I do desire the other for the other, whole and entire, male or female, because living means wanting everything that lives and wanting it alive. Castration. Let others toy with it. What's a desire originating from a lack? A pretty meagre desire.
>
> (Cixous, 1976 as cited in Frosh, 1994, p. 26).

If Horrocks and I are correct in our reading of Lacan, then there is something problematic and troubling for all psychotherapists, not just for Sexual Grounding practitioners, in the implied immutability of this state of affairs. Lacan was notably scathing about the (humanistic) therapies that began to emerge in the 1950s and that offered clients the possibility of enhanced and fulfilling lives by enabling them to feel whole in themselves rather than feeling a lack or deficiency, which we try to make up for in fantasy by desiring each other.

Lacan would assert we have to also separate ourselves from our environment, which includes the other human beings who occupy our world, in order to become aware of ourselves as separate beings, to develop an identity.[1] The problem is that, on the one hand, it *is* important that we, as therapists, recognise the depth and importance of the separation that exists in both in our own and in our clients' relationships with our environment.

On the other hand, it is also important to be able to experience ourselves as part of that environment again, not as an illusory wish to return to an undifferentiated state, which is how Lacan views it, but as part, and yet not part, of our environment. This is, I would argue, what relationships, and especially sexual relationships, are about. There is a tension between separation and connection and arguably, in the movement between the two, a concomitant vibration at work here.

In using the phrase 'part and yet not part', I want to imply a dynamic equilibrium between separation (individuality) and togetherness (unity). Dynamic equilibrium implies a freedom of movement between these states and it is the vibration that results from this movement that keeps our relationships, both with our environment and with each other, alive. Many, some would say all, of our problems, individual, relational, sexual, social and environmental can be attributed to a lack of understanding and acceptance of this equilibrium.

In accepting that the split nature of human beings and the classic Oedipal conflict together with its compromise resolution (see Lamb, 2017)[2] are both inevitable and immutable, psychoanalysis takes a very different route to that of SGT, but nevertheless provides a starting point for SGT to take both of these observable developmental phenomena in a more positive direction.

In his book on sexual difference Stephen Frosh (1994) acknowledges some of the weaknesses in the psychoanalytic position, especially its oculocentrism – the boy, apparently, fears castration because he *sees* that his sister doesn't have a penis and wonders what has happened to it. Of course, this is predicated on the idea that the boy couldn't simply ask his mother or father why his sister didn't have a penis and get an answer appropriate to his age. This would be the SGT position (see Chapter 5). However, Frosh, quoting Grosz (1990 as cited in Frosh, 1994), concludes that: 'The other sensory-perceptual organs would have confirmed the presence of a female organ instead of the absence of a male organ' (p. 30).

Describing her as 'the principal psychoanalyst of the physical' (Incorrectly in my view; I believe that title belongs to Wilhelm Reich!), Frosh brings Melanie Klein in at this point (Frosh, 1994, p. 30). Her contributions to the field of psychoanalysis, particularly her originating of object relations theory with its emphasis on projection and introjection, are certainly crucial, but again, there is a determinism in her writing that is troubling, especially her belief in both the death instinct and the infant's innate destructiveness.

Later object relations practitioners, especially D. W. Winnicott, see humanity in a much more positive light, using such concepts as 'the good-enough mother' (Winnicott, 1986) and especially developing the idea of maternal mirroring (Winnicott, 2000; Srinivasan, 2016), which relates very closely to Poppeliers' concept of 'sexual mirroring', which is one of the essential components of SGT.

One of the characteristics of Winnicott's work, which he shares with Wilhelm Reich, is that he takes a positive view of human beings and acknowledges the struggles involved in living fully and creatively in the world in which we find ourselves. I see both of these practitioners as examples of what we could call a 'bridge' between the psychodynamic and the humanistic territories. As I'm re-reading the work of both the traditional psychoanalytic writers and of these 'bridge' writers, I'm struck not only by the difference in their ways of looking at the world and the human beings who inhabit it, but also by *how* they write and, in particular, the picture I get of them as human beings behind their writing as I'm reading. I get pleasure from connecting to an author and what allows me to do this is the author's willingness and ability to share their vulnerability and passion with me (see the quote from Hélène Cixous, even though she's a philosopher rather than a psychotherapist, for an example of this style of writing).

Before I move on to look at the humanistic stream of therapy and its relationship to SGT, I would like to summarise this section.

As I have said in previous chapters, there's no doubt that SGT owes a lot to the pioneering work of the early psychoanalysts and especially to Freud. Privileging sexual energy (libido) as the life force of humanity and, initially at least, seeing disturbances of the libido as the origin of neurosis accords well with the belief system that underlies Willem Poppeliers' work.

However, when looked at from a 21st-century perspective, it's clear that Freud (together with his present-day traditional adherents) is imposing a medicalised, positivist framework onto the intricacies of human psychological development and experience, both the mysterious (to Freud) feminine and the insecure (which Freud arguably embodied) masculine. Freud was explicit about this in one of his later works, *Moses and Monotheism*, where he talks about the rise of patriarchy (a good thing in his view) saying:

> But this turning from the mother to the father points in addition to a victory of intellectuality over sensuality – that is an advance in civilisation, since maternity is proved by the senses while paternity is a hypothesis, based on an inference and a premise. Taking sides in this way with a thought process in preference to a sense perception has proved to be a momentous step.
>
> (Freud, 1939, p. 114)

In adopting the medicalised, positivist framework, Freud elevates the masculine quality of intellectual understanding, which requires distance/objectivity, over the feminine quality of just knowing, which requires connection and prizes subjectivity, and views the acceptance of the masculine superiority as an indication of psychic health. A rather shocking example of this is the Princess Marie

Bonaparte, a devoted disciple of Freud's. In an effort to experience a 'vaginal orgasm', which Freud had designated as superior to the clitoral orgasm, she is said to have had her clitoris surgically removed (Roazen, 1992).

Since one of the central tenets of SGT is the developmental balancing of masculinity and femininity at an internal level, effectively internalising both of our parents, and exploring this at a bodily level, there's clearly a contradiction between the SGT and psychoanalytic perspectives on, and therefore ways of working with, the human condition. The first is about balance and harmony and the second is about submission and control. For the present, and in the interest of balance, the best thing we can do is to express our debt of gratitude to Freud for his pioneering work in the field of psychosexual therapy and at the same time follow the developments of his work that make intuitive sense to us at a body level.

Another way of looking at this would be to say that there is much common language between psychoanalysis and SGT, both in their diagnostic terms and in the vocabulary used to describe the unconscious processes that both disciplines recognise. What they see as important and, indeed, *possible* in the work they do with clients/patients is, however, markedly different.

Moving on to look at the humanistic stream of psychotherapy, I want to acknowledge that this stream is as broad and diverse as the psychodynamic. For example, my own experience of becoming an accredited psychotherapist is that practitioners such as myself, who have trained in Reichian and bioenergetic psychotherapy, can be accredited in the UK by the United Kingdom Association of Humanistic Psychology Practitioners, even though both of these models incorporate a considerable degree of psychoanalytic influence.

Humanistic psychotherapy, which is epitomised in the work of Carl Rogers, Fritz Perls and Eric Berne et al., is characterised, as its name suggests, by its belief in humanity. To be more precise, the belief is that human beings and their impulses, drives and desires are essentially, in the literal sense of that word, healthy and life-enhancing. Human beings are inherently creative and naturally move towards experiences that give them the possibility of fulfilment, which is our birthright. There is nothing wrong, negative or intrinsically evil about a newborn infant who, given appropriate responses from their environment, will strive towards this self-fulfilment.

The roots of humanism, the philosophical system which shares the beliefs described above, probably go back to the days of the Enlightenment in the late 17th and 18th century as a reaction to Catholicism and Calvinism, both of which embrace the idea of original sin, which I mentioned earlier in Part 1. I'm not putting myself forward as an English scholar, but I very much doubt that Blake (I'm thinking about his *Songs of Innocence and Experience* here) and the Romantic poets who were writing at about that time would disagree with many of the beliefs of SGT, particularly about childhood innocence (Blake, 2017), sexual freedom and liberation.

In a similar way, humanistic psychology was developed in response to what Carl Rogers, for example, saw as the two prevalent and equally, for their own reasons, pessimistic streams of psychology and psychotherapy he encountered, i.e. psychoanalysis and behaviourism. The emphasis in both of these models of therapy, especially in America in Rogers' time, was on control by the therapist. In response, Carl Rogers' emphasis was on re-empowering the client (the first step was to use the word 'client' rather than 'patient'), and he did this by putting the client at the centre of the therapeutic relationship (Rogers, 1976). This has a resonance with Willem Poppeliers' emphasis on putting the child (both real children and inner children) at the centre of the work in SGT. This will become apparent in Part 3.

It's clear from the above that Carl Rogers' approach, known as Person Centred Therapy, has a lot in common with some of the core beliefs of SGT. The ideas around innocence and the natural tendency towards self-fulfilment accord well with the goals that SGT aims to support in clients. Seeing the purpose of therapy as enabling the client to work towards their own fulfilment (Rogers calls this the actualising tendency) rather than simply curing their presenting problems is also common to both models.

The prizing of the therapeutic relationship is another common thread, even though in SGT the healing relationships are mostly between the client and the person or persons who are re-enacting their parents rather than between therapist and client. Carl Rogers' 'Core Conditions' (unconditional positive regard for the client, empathy and congruence) are the backbone of most therapists' practice and SGT therapists are no exception to this.

The most obvious difference between the two models is that the person-centred approach seems to leave out sex altogether. A Google search for 'Sexuality in the work of Carl Rogers' brought up some interesting articles on the use of person-centred techniques with sexual minorities and survivors of sexual abuse but nothing at all on the place of sexuality in his actual work. I suspect that, again, this comes down to an issue of fear and control. Carl Rogers wanted to liberate human creativity and potential and, given the way that the existing therapies were practised in America at that time, this was clearly a good thing and was well received by the post-war American generation – the baby boomers. (On a personal note, it was reading Carl Rogers' book on encounter groups (Rogers, 1970) that set me off on the road to becoming both a therapist and the person I am today). However, explicitly including sexuality at the same time as acknowledging the power and importance of the client's relationship with the therapist and not directing or controlling this would perhaps have been just too challenging, both to person centred therapists and to the society in which they were practising. One only has to think about the furore caused when Brian Thorne published his article, 'Beyond the Core Conditions', to see how this disturbed the person-centred community (Dryden, 1987).

Whilst one might expect the work of Fritz Perls, influenced as he was by Reich, to be more explicitly centred on sexual fulfilment, it is remarkably absent from Gestalt Therapy. It is true that there is more emphasis on the body and bodily experience of feelings in Gestalt Therapy than in person-centred work, but sexuality isn't explicitly worked with. Thinking about Perls himself, he *is* explicit that he, to use a psychoanalytic term, 'acts out his erotic counter-transference' with his female clients rather than working on it as a therapeutic issue (Perls, 1969). Since then, as Leanne O'Shea (2000) observes in an article in the *Gestalt Review*, Gestalt therapists and writers have been so careful to avoid being linked with Perls' behaviour that they tend to avoid sexuality, especially when it arises in the therapeutic relationship itself.

In SGT there is a focus on the inner child and also on our internalised parents, and this has resonances with Eric Berne's Transactional Analysis (TA). In my own practice, especially with couples, I find this connection useful in that many of my clients have come across TA and so the basic language is familiar to them. However, the way in which SGT focuses on and uses these concepts, which actually has more in common with the work of Hal and Sidra Stone's voice dialogue work (Stone & Stone, 2011), is different to how they are used in TA.

Transactional Analysis, by definition, concerns itself with the analysis of transactions between two potentially equal human beings and how these become distorted as a result of the positions, or ego states, that the participants adopt. There is also a focus on the games that are involved in the adoption of the different ego states.

SGT focuses on what the child in us didn't get at an appropriate stage of psychosexual development, e.g., sexual mirroring. This missing affirmation and regulation clearly distorts our adult sexual relationships. SGT works with this by using exercises and structures which allow participants to re-experience the stage of psychosexual development at which the appropriate responses from parents were missing and to replay the crucial scenes in a much more positive way using fellow participants as parents. In effect, when we do this, we are 'rewriting our script'. This is a concept which is also central to TA, but there are two important differences.

Firstly, SGT works with the body and the change of script works not only with language but also with touch, sight, sound and sometimes smell. This means that it's not only the script that changes but also, as in other body therapies such as Bioenergetics, the visceral, muscular and sensory experience. Ultimately, this means that the brain is effectively re-programmed at a deep level and new neural connections being forged according to Hebb's law, 'Neurons that fire together wire together' (Hebb, 1949).

Secondly, in TA the scripts are usually (unconscious) decisions, taken in early childhood, in response to injunctions and counter-injunctions from parents and other significant figures. Examples of injunctions are:

Don't be needy
Don't be childish
Don't feel

Don't grow up
Etc.

Examples of counter-injunctions are:

Be perfect
Please me
Try hard
Be strong for me
Etc.

(see Newton, 2018)

As can be seen from the above examples, these scripts only have one character, that of the internalised (I don't think Berne used that term) parent. This is very different to the scripts in SGT. In the structures of SGT, there are usually at least three characters – the participant, their 'mother' and their 'father'. It is also not uncommon to include grandparents and other significant family members in these structures. Another way of describing the process in SGT is 'rewriting the story'. This was certainly my own experience as a participant. Although sexuality *may* be a part of a client's script and there are very likely to be injunctions and counter-injunctions on the subject in most client's psyches, it doesn't seem to feature specifically in the TA literature so that unless the client is specifically wanting to work on that aspect of their life, it is unlikely to be part of the work.

The idea of rewriting our story leads me to the cognitive and behavioural stream of therapy. Certainly, in Cognitive Behavioural Therapy (CBT), rewriting and re-interpreting experiences is a significant feature of the work and is therefore a connection with SGT. The idea of re-programming, which I mentioned earlier, would also be familiar to a CBT therapist. The two differences, which are significant, are firstly that CBT has a strong emphasis on control, both the therapist's control of the therapeutic process and also the goal of getting the client 'back in control' of their feelings and eradicating their uncomfortable symptoms. Secondly, CBT, as the name suggests, is mostly carried out at a conscious verbal level, whereas SGT is very much focussed on unconscious patterns that are embodied.

Sexuality is not explicitly included in CBT, but it isn't totally excluded either. Since the driving purpose of CBT is explicitly the reduction of symptoms, then the work a CBT therapist will offer to a client who presents with a psychosexual issue will be very different from the SGT approach. Nevertheless, it's clear from the work we do in SGT that the way we think about ourselves as sexual beings has a significant effect on our experience of sexuality and relationships. Changing this is certainly going to be beneficial, the difference being that, in SGT, these cognitive changes are underpinned and reinforced by embodied and relational experience.

As can be seen from the brief exploration above, SGT has important connections with all three of the main streams of psychotherapy. This can give us a common language when talking to professional colleagues. It seems to me that the differences mostly centre on control and sexuality.

The psychodynamic stream includes sexuality but sees psychic health as a state where the potentially chaotic impulses of the id are controlled by the superego in the service of the ego. The cognitive behavioural stream has a lot of focus on control, both the therapist's and the client's, and this includes the way in which sexual and psychosexual issues are worked with. The humanistic stream believes much more in human potential and is therefore much less interested in control but, perhaps because of the perceived danger of 'uncontrolled' sexuality, leaves psychosexual issues out of its work. One of the unique features of SGT is that it isn't focused on control (although there is an emphasis on regulation, both in the work itself and in the aims of the therapy[3]), but it also explicitly includes sexuality and psychosexual development as primary features of the work.

Its aim is to liberate sexual energy and impulses from what are often self-imposed restrictions that have a debilitating effect on all aspects of clients' lives and, at the same time, to do this in a regulated environment which supports the development of self-regulation.

Another significant difference between SGT and most other forms of mainstream psychotherapy is that, whilst SGT begins, as to some extent all forms of psychotherapy do, by addressing the issues that have arisen for clients in their childhood and that are affecting their life in the present, it continues through the stages of maturation and projects the client into the future to work on their aging process and even their death.

SGT is not unique in this respect. Erik Erikson worked with a series of 'life crises', which extended from earliest childhood up to the 1960s and beyond (see Erikson, 1963) and there is some relationship between Erikson's life stages and the 'tasks' which he assigns to them (e.g., the task in adolescence is to discover one's identity) and the stages in SGT. The difference is that, for Willem Poppeliers, the focus is on sexuality and how it is lived and experienced at each stage.

Gail Sheehy (1977) was also interested in emotional development across the lifespan. Her stages, mostly decades, are more specific than Erikson's but are also much more focussed on life in general than those used in SGT.

In this chapter, I've presented a picture of how SGT fits in with the three main streams of psychotherapy. One way of framing this would be to say that it integrates features from all of these streams and could therefore be described as an 'integrative' therapy. However, most therapists would describe their work in this way and the term doesn't really tell us that much. A more daring conclusion we could draw is that, because of its unique combination of freedom, depth and working specifically with sexuality and regulation, SGT doesn't really fit in with any of the conventional models of psychotherapy.

Notes

1 See Erikson's stages of psychosocial development where the world of the child expands from the mother to the parents, to the family, school, society and finally humanity in general (Erikson, 1963).

2 In this article I contrast the traditional psychoanalytic version of what happens at the Oedipal stage of development – the child's incestuous longing to possess and have sex with the parent of the opposite sex, which, under threat of castration, has to be renounced and the threatening power, usually of the parent of the same sex, internalised as the superego – with Willem Poppeliers' version of what could happen at this stage with well-adjusted and regulated parents.

3 One question that frequently arises during the coursework is about the difference between control and regulation. There are different ways of thinking about this. The first is to take a classic example of the boy who wants to show his genitals to his parents. According to the principles of SGT, this is a natural and innocent impulse that merits a positive response, which is the beginning of regulation. A 'control' response, which could either come from the parents' own embarrassment or from their concern that, if they give a positive response, the boy would learn that exposing his genitals is a good thing and do it again in all sorts of inappropriate situations, would be to discipline the boy and make him feel bad for exposing himself.

The 'regulation' response, having begun by giving a positive response to the boy's penis, would be to wait and see if he started to show it in inappropriate situations – at school or to strangers. If this were to happen, and SGT theory suggests that it is less likely rather than more likely to happen if the boy gets a positive response from his parents because he then has no need to receive affirmation because he's already had it, it is clearly important to explain to the boy that, although you don't believe he's done anything wrong, it's either inappropriate, or in some cases dangerous, to show your genitals outside the family.

Another more subtle way of thinking about the difference between control and regulation is that the way of helping children develop self-regulation is by encouraging them to trust themselves. This encourages them to become aware of, sensitive to and connected with themselves. From this position they begin to become aware of, sensitive to and connected with others and with their environment. Self-regulation is the inevitable result of such awareness, which we could also refer to as empathy.

References

Blake, W. (2017). *Songs of innocence and experience*. London: Penguin.

Dryden, W. (1987). *Key cases in psychotherapy*. London: Croom Publishers.

Erikson, E. (1963). *Childhood and society*. New York: W. W. Norton & Co.

Freud, S. (1939). *Moses and monotheism*. London: Hogarth Press.

Freud, S. (1969). *The psychopathology of everyday life*. London: Ernest Benn Ltd.

Frosh, S. (1994). *Sexual difference: Masculinity and psychoanalysis*. London: Routledge.

Hebb, D. O. (1949). *The organisation of behaviour*. New York: Wiley & Sons.

Horrocks, R. (1997). *An introduction to the study of sexuality*. Basingstoke: MacMillan.

Lamb, G. (2017). 'Beyond Oedipus'. Available at: http://www.geoff-lamb-psycho therapist.com/article-beyond-oedipus.html

Newton, C. (2018). 'Transactional analysis – Part III: The scripts we follow'. Available at: http://www.clairenewton.co.za/my-articles/transactional-analysis-part-iii-the-scripts-we-follow.html

O'Shea, L. (2000). 'Sexuality: Old struggles, new Challenges'. *Gestalt Review*, 4(1), 8–25.

Perls, F. (1969). *In and out the garbage pail*. New York: Gestalt Journal Press.

Roazen, P. (1992). *Freud and his followers*. New York: Da Capo Press.

Rogers, C. (1970). *On encounter groups*. New York: Harper Collins.

Rogers, C. (1976). *Client centred therapy*. London: Constable.

Rowan, J. (2005). *The future of training in psychotherapy and counselling*. London: Routledge.

Sheehy, G. (1977). *Passages*. London: Dutton Books.

Srinivasan, S. K. (2016). Donald Winnicott and the mirroring function. Clinical notes series [PowerPoint slides]. SlideShare. Available at: https://www.slideshare.net/Shiva KumarSrinivasan/donald-winnicott-on-the-mirroring-function

Stone, H., & Stone, S. (2011). *Embracing ourselves*. New York: New World.

Winnicott, D. W. (1986). *Home is where we start from*. London: Pelican.

Winnicott, D. W. (2000). *The child, the family and the outside world*. London: Penguin.

World Health Organization (WHO). (2006). *Defining sexual health: Report of a technical consultation on sexual health 28–31 January 2002, Geneva*. Geneva: WHO. Available at: https://www.who.int/reproductivehealth/publications/sexual_health/defining_sexua l_health.pdf

Chapter 4

Non-mainstream ways of working with sexuality and sexual issues

Up to now, in this part of the book, I have drawn extensively on my experience of psychotherapy as a client, practitioner and trainer. In this chapter, I will be commenting from the position of an outside observer and sometime participant. Whilst the position I am commenting from is necessarily less informed than that in the preceding chapter, I believe that it is important to include other approaches since these are very often participants' route into Sexual Grounding Therapy (SGT) and, in some cases, have been influential on its development. For example, the masculine and feminine breathing (the man imagining himself breathing in through his heart and out through his genitals and the woman doing the opposite), which forms part of the exercises in Coursework 1 of SGT, is derived from tantric principles, as I shall explain in the section of this chapter that focusses on Tantra. Whether they refer to themselves as 'therapy' or not, and many don't, the non-mainstream ways of working with sexuality are increasingly where people turn when they are experiencing difficulties.

The common factor, which SGT shares with all of the non-mainstream ways of working with sexuality that I'm going to look at, is that they seem to be working towards the similar goal of supporting their clients in their pursuit of intimate and fulfilling sexual relationships. How they do this, how they view sexuality and how they think about what prevents human beings from achieving this goal is where the differences with SGT lie. In this chapter I'm going to focus on Pelvic-Heart Integration (PHI), Tantra, sex coaching and Somatic Sex Education/Sexological Bodywork.

Pelvic-Heart Integration

The non-mainstream therapy that is most similar to SGT is Pelvic-Heart Integration (PHI). This, of course, is not surprising since its founder, Jack Painter, worked in close collaboration with Willem Poppeliers. My account of PHI is based on an interview with Dirk Marivoet on 18 April, 2018 and on some written material that he was kind enough to recently send me.

The similarities PHI shares with SGT are that it works across the whole lifespan, includes work with participants role-playing ideal parents, uses physical movement and breathing to enable participants to make contact with feelings, emphasises the importance of mirroring and, it seems, has little written about it and is not very widespread. The language used to describe the work also has many similarities. There is a lot of emphasis on the balance between masculine and feminine inside the individual and also on how sexuality is lived and experienced at different stages of psychosexual development (Renner & Marivoet, 2020).

One difference from SGT is that PHI does a lot of work with pre-genital (pre-Oedipal) issues, modelling itself quite closely on Alexander Lowen's character structures and using a specific breathing for each, e.g., the 'secure' breath for the schizoid structure (Lowen, 1959).[1] There seems to be a strong connection between this work and bioenergetics, with a lot of hands on work on the part of the therapist designed to enable breathing to be full and relaxed by using deep tissue massage. The assumption, in Jack Painter's article on his natural energetic cycle (Painter, 2007), seems to be that most clients will have some kind of disturbance to their breathing and energy circulation and that these will need to be worked through with the assistance of a therapist.

Another difference between PHI and SGT is that PHI is delivered both as an individual therapy and a group therapy, the latter being also the route for the training of practitioners, which takes approximately three years. Although psychotherapy is referred to on the website, PHI doesn't specifically define itself as a psychotherapy even though its practitioners may be therapeutically qualified in their own right before embarking on the training.

Although there are sometimes spiritual implications to some of the SGT concepts (e.g., Willem Poppeliers' use of the word 'paradise' (see Chapter 10), and it is certainly true that some SGT practitioners hold their own spiritual beliefs which inform their work, spirituality isn't specifically included in SGT theory. It is very much part of the theory and aims of PHI, the final breaths in the cycle of nine moving beyond Lowen's character structures into the cosmic realm.[2]

My overall and, I have to acknowledge, subjective impression of this work is that it is very systematic. There is much to recommend it and, not altogether surprisingly, considerable common language between it and SGT. I had a concern, both as a Sexual Grounding therapist and also as an ex-counselling trainer, about the blurring between the group therapy and the therapeutic training and also about its brevity and the fact that no previous therapeutic qualifications are required before admission to the training programme. I was also not clear, either in my reading or in my conversation with Marivoet, how the erotic transference/counter-transference would be handled in one to one PHI work. In relation to the split between Painter and Poppeliers, Marivoet alluded, in our Skype conversation, to a 'clash of personalities', but neither of us mentioned boundaries, either in the past or in the present functioning of PHI. Nevertheless, I was left with the impression that there could be some useful dialogue between practitioners of both disciplines (there are actually a few SGT practitioners who have been trained in, and still practise, PHI) even though the ways of working have diverged irreconcilably.

Tantra

My knowledge of Tantra is limited to personal experiences and brief reading. I'm very aware of its considerable history and teachings, which I won't be referring to, but I'm very interested, and will focus on, its relationship with SGT. My experience of, and reading about, Tantra suggest that the focus on the flow of sexual energy in the body and the connection between heart and genitals represents an immediate common ground with SGT. Masculine and feminine principles and their relationship with each other, internally and externally, are also common features of both disciplines. Above all, in (re)-uniting spirituality and sexuality, Tantra goes some way to addressing the issues of religious control I discussed in Chapter 1, bringing energy and freedom back into sexual expression and experience within an overall spiritual context. This is something which has been a problem for the Abrahamic and patriarchal religions, and in Western culture generally, for millennia.

My observation and understanding is that Tantra, whilst having the objective of freeing the flow of sexual energy in the body, doesn't concern itself much with the origins of the blocks to the flow of that energy. The idea of 'sexual healing' certainly is part of modern Tantra (Anand, 1989; Richardson, 2003), but the healing seems to take place in the present. I was also interested to discover that Margo Anand (1989) acknowledges that some of the healing exercises she uses are derived from Jack Painter's work.

Diana Richardson's approach is particularly interesting from a therapeutic perspective and *Tantric Love: Feeling vs Emotion* epitomises the healing aspect of her work (Richardson, 2010). Drawing on the writings of spiritual teachers such as Eckhart Tolle (2006) and Don Miguel Ruiz (1997) as well as Marshall's Non-violent Communication Theory (Rosenberg, 2003), Richardson's work resonates closely with my own couplework training and practice, especially in its recommendations to couples who get involved in intractable arguments and emotional impasses. The idea that one partner will eventually be convinced by the rightness of the other's perspective, together with the whole idea of right and wrong in the context of a relationship, is seriously challenged, and this, when I came across it, brought back echoes of my own couple training with Nick Duffell and Helena Løvendal (Duffel & Løvendal, 2006).

However, whilst it sensitively acknowledges in some detail the role of childhood experience in all kinds of contemporary psychosexual difficulty, especially early trauma, Richardson's work differs from SGT in that parents, transferentially or otherwise, are not involved in the process of healing. It's very much about self-help, by which I mean the couple each taking responsibility for their own process and their own needs, which can be empowering and transformational in itself but is different from the SGT approach.

Richardson focuses practically and directly on enhancing couples' lovemaking experience. This has two consequences. The first is that the work is mostly orientated towards couples, although some of Richardson's writing, especially that for women, is aimed at individuals. As well as offering her couples' programme with her partner Michael, she also offers tantric retreats for women under the title 'Time for Femininity'. Richardson chooses to focus her work on couples because, as she puts it, 'That is how I learned, in a couple…' (Richardson, personal communication, 2020). The second consequence is that her work, both written and experiential, contains exercises and meditations with detailed instructions, such as those she describes in her books *Slow Sex* and *The Heart of Tantric Sex* (Richardson, 2011; 2003), which are designed to enable, for example, both partners to be fully present when making love. These exercises, concerning presence and contact, are combined with practical input on lovemaking itself, which is both helpful and inspiring.

Whilst SGT welcomes couples who wish to attend the coursework, it is primarily focussed on participants' individual experience of themselves as developing sexual beings and how *this* experience, which has often been negative in real life, can be healed in a way which will feed through into their relationships. In effect, a couple attending the SGT programme does so as two individuals, each working on their own psychosexual developmental issues. Clearly, this work will have an effect on their relationship, but this is not the focus of the work itself. Individuals *do* present relationship difficulties in the coursework, especially in the process work, and participants report considerable improvement, not to say transformation, in their relationships as a result of their participation in the SGT programme; however, the focus of the work is not on couple relationships or on lovemaking itself. That said, there is some input, in SGT, about genitals being organs of contact and connection rather than focussing on orgasm as a discharge of energy, and this is one important similarity with Diana Richardson's tantric approach.

Like the mainstream psychotherapies I described in Chapter 3, Tantra is a broad field and there is considerable variation in how it is taught. One area where I have observed differences, mostly in conversations with fellow sexuality professionals, is in the area of boundaries. In its aim of helping people to free themselves from the socially imposed inhibitions, which I've already written about and which is a broadly shared aim with SGT, there is sometimes a tendency in Tantra to be less concerned about sexual boundaries. I have to say I don't have direct experience of this myself and, on the contrary, my experience with Diana and Michael Richardson was exemplary in this respect.

In researching this book, I spoke with my colleague, Notburga Fischer who, as well as being an experienced SGT trainer, also has a wealth of experience in the field of Tantra. She was of the opinion that, whilst the creation of the 'love temple', a free space where participants can explore their impulses, was a liberating aspect of some modern Tantra courses, there was also a danger that participants who were in committed relationships could put those relationships at risk by 'acting out' the experimentation phase behaviours (which belong to the puberty/adolescence stage which I will describe in Chapter 6) with a succession of different partners. In effect, whilst the workshop leaders occupy the role of permission-giving parents who are perhaps unlike the repressive parents who participants may have experienced in real life, there is no recognition or processing of the transference involved. This, she believes, can make the liberating experience difficult to integrate into real life.

Fischer also had a concern that people who had experienced sexual abuse or unclear sexual boundaries in their formative years would be attracted to Tantra as a way of healing the wounds caused by these experiences. This is understandable, but she felt that there was a strong possibility that they would also take these abusive patterns into their tantric experience. Not being able to feel their own boundaries and to say 'no' at an appropriate moment could lead to the re-stimulation of old wounds rather than the healing they were looking for (N. Fischer, personal communication, 2020).

One way of thinking about this, without becoming overcritical of other practitioners' work, is to recognise that the sexual energy we're all working with is extremely powerful. The fact that this energy has been repressed for as long as it has, in both the individual and society, means that, when released, it can easily emerge in an unregulated way. This is consistent with Reichian theory and was one of the problems that he encountered with the (psychoanalytic) establishment and were arguably the cause of his prosecution by the American authorities. Criticisms of his liberated approach to sex were often based, not so much on what Reich and his immediate followers either did themselves or encouraged in others, but on how individuals with a limited understanding of his work believed they were allowed to behave sexually as followers of his philosophy. To be fair, Reich himself wasn't overconcerned with these criticisms and, although he commented on them later in his life in *Listen Little Man* (Reich, 1974), he wasn't as scrupulous about correcting these misinterpretations of his beliefs as he could have been. I suspect it is much the same with Tantra.

It is also a possibility that some Tantra practitioners take a similar view to Jack Painter (see Chapter 2) – that participants are able, as adults, to make their own decisions about where their sexual boundaries are and can take care of these in workshop situations without needing them to be imposed from the outside. For this reason, some people, particularly when they come to the work from a Tantra background, can experience the carefully considered guidelines we use in SGT, which we see as necessary in an environment where participants are exploring vulnerable areas of their lives, as being repressive and controlling.[3]

Sex coaching

My research into sex coaching has been mostly internet-based, supplemented by collegial discussions with members of Sexuality Professionals UK, a support/networking group I joined just over a year ago. The word 'coaching', in a sports context, has been around for many years and refers to the encouragement, training and general all-round management of sportsmen/women or teams. More recently, coaching has emerged as a relative of psychotherapy and counselling, where it has the characteristic of being more directive with homework, assignments, action plans, measurable goals, etc.

Sex coaching seems to share many of these characteristics, although the term covers a broad range of practitioners each of whom has their own individual definition of what their work involves. Thus, according to the World Association of Sex Coaches website, coaches accredited by that organisation are allowed to use 'healing and appropriate touch' in the course of their work although some of the coaches whose websites I visited were clear that they did not do so (Valentine-Chase, 2020; Rowett, 2018).

This quote by Lucy Rowett, the founder and organiser of Sexuality Professionals UK, from her Sex Coaching website, gives a flavour of what the work involves:

> Sessions consist of intuitive guidance, emotional releasing, trying different techniques, personalized sex education and home assignments. It's a co-creation between you and me to help you achieve your sex and relationship goals. I'll be your guide and cheerleader, and expect me to hold you accountable to your goals! You may find some uncomfortable emotions coming up, but this part of the process.
>
> (Rowett, 2018)

Rowett is careful to distinguish her work from psychotherapy and states that she will refer on to a therapist if she believes it's in the client's interest (Rowett, 2018).

The similarities with SGT are that the overall goal is liberating clients from the shame they may have associated with sexuality and helping them to create and sustain intimate and fulfilling sexual relationships. Sex coaching acknowledges that previous (childhood) experiences will probably be having a deleterious effect on clients' current sex lives, but it doesn't make these the focus of the work. Instead, it seeks to replace these negative experiences and thoughts with more positive goals. Although most sex coaches would endorse the idea of sex being part of the rest of a client's life and many coaches do pay attention to relationships and intimacy, the focus of the work seems to be on the (mechanics of) sex itself rather than, as in SGT, sex as part of the client's relationship with their fellow human beings, especially parents and lovers, and with their environment.

Somatic Sex Education

I'm including Sexological Bodywork/Somatic Sex Education because, whilst they are explicitly 'hands on' in the work they do, they also have a very strict code of ethics and are clearly aiming at the same combination of freedom and regulation as SGT. Their professional body, The Association of Somatic and Integrative Sexologists (ASIS), which accredits a broad cross-section of sexuality practitioners, is also welcoming to Sexual Grounding therapists and trainers.

The similarities with SGT seem to be that Somatic Sex Education works, as its name suggests, with sexual energy at a body level and has the goal of removing the blocks associated with childhood sex-negative experiences, which get in the way of a satisfying and intimate experience and expression of our sexuality.

I am basing this section on my reading (Jesse, 2016; 2017; Pelmas, 2017), my own brief experience of individual Somatic Sex Education sessions with certified sexological bodyworker, Jem Ayres, and a very useful conversation with Kian De La Cour and Katie Sarra who have developed and deliver the UK & Ireland Somatic Sex Education professional trainings and were kind enough to take the time to meet with me at the Sea School of Embodiment in Dawlish.

As its title suggests, the work, described as 'education', has a focus on coaching. Practitioners have the scope of practice to include touch, including genital touch, if appropriate. They also learn non-tactile methods of facilitating embodied enquiry, such as body focusing and Clean Language, a style of working with metaphor and clarifying questions developed by David Grove in the 1980s (Wilson, 2017). Like SGT, Somatic Sex Education may involve (appropriate)[4] nudity on the part of the client (student), the ethics specifying that the educator remains clothed at all times, with erotic touch being strictly 'one-way'.

The process of the 'education' in my personal experience, although it recognises the importance of childhood issues, especially of trauma and/or neglect, is mostly based in the present and the future. It is therefore described as being a trauma-informed rather than trauma-focussed modality. Having said that, I imagine that, if material had come up for me that I needed to talk about, offload feelings about or get support with in my work with Jem Ayres, there would certainly have been space for this. I was aware that I didn't choose to fill in all of the sections on her comprehensive intake form, which offered space to highlight these kinds of issues had I felt I needed to include them in the work.

I had clearly done a lot of work on myself, specifically focussed on the issues of childhood, so I didn't feel a strong need to explore these further in this context and so was comfortable with the massage, exercises and meditations. These were both useful and powerful, but, from this experience and my reading and discussions, I gained the impression that transference and counter-transference are not a particular aspect of this work that is given a lot of attention.

One way in which transference is managed in Somatic Sex Education is that the touch, as well as being one-way, is very much in the control of the client, who is supported in asking for the kind of touch he/she wants and its location on the body. Many Somatic Sex Educators use Betty Martin's 'Wheel of Consent' as a tool in their work (Martin, 2020) both as a means of regulating the sessions and as a tool to pass onto their clients. All of this creates a safety for the client and is at the same time empowering for them, both in the sessions and in the rest of their lives. However, an important difference with SGT is that in SGT touch is normally exchanged between the client and a transferential/role-playing parent, always a fellow group member and never the therapist/trainer, again with consent being sought and given. This means that any issues or blocks that may arise and that have to do with past experience can be processed by the client in the transference (see Chapter 10).

The processing of issues and blocks that arise transferentially is the purpose of the work in SGT. In Somatic Sex Education, the purpose of the work is to 'restore the client's capacity for interroception so that they can better be in choice about self-regulating their arousal and being curious about sensation rather than stuck in old habits' (K. De La Cour, personal communication, 2020).[5] The purpose of the touch is often, but not always, for the client to allow themselves to experience pleasure in the touch itself, whereas, in SGT, where touch is used, it is primarily for the purpose of recognition and affirmation.

As a practitioner, I'm not sure if I would feel comfortable with the level of intimate contact involved in Sexological Bodywork/Somatic Sex Education. In my practice as an individual therapist, which is the context where I work most directly with transference and counter-transference, it's important for me to know who I am in my interactions with my clients, whether I'm their father, mother, lover, etc. This is particularly important when it comes to touch. I rarely use touch in my practice these days (my original training in Bioenergetics was quite hands on, but then the purpose of the touch was to help the client free up their energy blocks). These days I work quite relationally and it's important for me to be clear about the nature of the relationship.

In my practice as an SGT therapist and trainer, my role is to oversee the transference/counter-transference interaction between participants; in the process work (see Part 3), some people have compared this to being a theatre or film director. In the more formal structures, the framework of the structure has the function of establishing who is who in whatever contact is happening between participants. In process work, I find myself feeding participants lines like, 'What happens in your body, as a father, when your daughter talks to you about her boyfriend?' The purpose of this is to keep them aware of the role-play relationship, especially at a body level, which also has the effect of keeping the relationship real. The important thing is that everyone knows who they are in relation to each other.

From my experience and research, it seems that the relationship is thought of, in Sexological Bodywork/Somatic Sex Education, as being between professional and client. Kian de la Cour clarified the relationship as follows:

> We see it as coach and coachee, meeting non-hierarchically. I think it is important to state that [Somatic Sex Education] is not therapy. We explicitly encourage practitioners to be non-evaluative and often non-directive. We are not treating a client, we are facilitating the student's exploration and eliciting the student's innate knowledge of self. As practitioners of

Sexological Bodywork, we aim to embody Carl Rogers' core conditions of counselling of:

1   Congruence (genuineness)
2   Unconditional positive regard (U.P.R.) and acceptance
3   Accurate empathic understanding.
                        (K. De La Cour, personal communication, 2020)

Whilst, as SGT practitioners, we would certainly see ourselves as supporting participants' innate body wisdom and, as I've said in Chapter 3 of this part of the book, would also hope to embody Carl Rogers' core conditions, we are acutely aware, in our work, of unconscious process, especially erotic transference and counter-transference, which we work with specifically and deliberately as part of the healing process.

I'm aware that there may well be a depth in the training of Somatic Sex Educators that I've been unable to perceive in my research and that could address the discomfort I've explored above. I can definitely see some important connections between their work and what we're trying to achieve in SGT. I'm also aware that, in SGT, we're usually most interested in healing past wounds that get in the way of full sexual experience and expression, and, as a result, we don't focus much on the mechanics of sexual experience, contact and pleasure. Somatic Sex Education clearly does. There could certainly be some room for dialogue here and both disciplines could potentially learn from each other.

As I said at the beginning of Part 2, there is a lot of sexual distress in the world, and, in response to this, there are many professionals who are making themselves available to help. Mainstream psychotherapy doesn't seem to be addressing psychosexual issues as effectively as it might for the reasons I've explored in Chapter 3, and so alternatives are being developed (in some cases revived) and are becoming more popular. I have explored the connections with, and differences between, SGT and both the mainstream and non-mainstream models of working with sexuality. One common factor with all of the non-mainstream approaches, with the exception of PHI, is that the non-mainstream models have a direct focus on clients' sexuality as experienced in the present and independent of parental influence whereas SGT and PHI see sexuality in a developmental context and use the relationship with parents as part of the exploration and healing. All of the models have some connection with SGT and one of our decisions in the future will be what we want to do with these connections. This will be explored in the final section of this book.

Notes

1 Alexander Lowen, building on Reich's work with character, divides human psychological development into a series of 'character structures': physical, behavioural and energetic characteristics dependent on the developmental stage at which the emotional disturbance (to the optimal course of human development) occurred. The schizoid structure is thought to relate to disturbance at the neonatal stage of development.
2 Jack Painter works with a cycle of nine breaths, some of which he describes in his book, which is available online. See: https://icpit.org/jack-painters-natural-energetic-cycle/
3 Of course, the fact that the revival of interest in Tantra has its roots in the work of Osho/Sri Rajneesh might be a factor here. When I was doing my training in the late 1970s and early 1980s in London, his organisation certainly seemed, from the outside, to have boundaries that were very different from those I was learning in my training. I don't have enough direct experience or knowledge of his work to be able to make a definitive connection here, although I did have conversations with some of his followers who came to some of the Bioenergetic workshops I was involved in at that time in which it was suggested that the boundaries within which we operated were over-strict. It is worth noting that, however his work may have been interpreted, when Osho talks about Tantra, he is not only talking about sex but also offering a new perspective on the whole of life, free of conditioning and repression. In this respect, his teaching is very much in tune with the objectives of SGT.
4 'Appropriate nudity' in SGT means that, subject to a detailed set of guidelines that all participants are required to sign before commencing the coursework and where the purpose of an exercise, process or structure requires it, nudity is involved in the work (see Chapter 12).
5 Interoception can be defined as 'being aware of internal body sensations'.

References

Anand, M. (1989). *The art of sexual ecstasy*. New York: Penguin Putnam Inc.

Duffell, N., & Løvendal-Duffell, H. (2006). *Love, sex and the dangers of intimacy*. London: Harper Collins.

Jesse, C. (2016). *Science for sexual happiness*. Salt Spring Island, BC: Erospirit.

Jesse, C. (2017). *Healers on the edge*. Salt Spring Island, BC: Erospirit.

Lowen, A. (1959). *The language of the body*. New York: Collier Paperbacks.

Martin, B. (2020). 'The wheel of consent'. Available at: www.bettymartin.org/videos

Painter, J. (2007). 'Jack Painter's "natural energetic cycle"'. Gent: International Community of Psychocorporal (Bodymind) Integration Trainers and Practitioners. Available at: http s://icpit.org/jack-painters-natural-energetic-cycle/

Pelmas, C. (2017). *Trauma: A practical guide to working with body and soul*. Scotts Valley, CA: CreateSpace Independent Publishing Platform.

Renner, E., & Marivoet, D. (2020). 'Pelvic-Heart integration'. Available at: https://www. pelvic-heart-integration.eu/pelvic-heart-integration-levels-masculine-feminine/

Reich, W. (1974). *Listen little man*. London: Pelican.

Richardson, D. (2003). *The heart of tantric sex*. London: O-Books.

Richardson, D. (2010). *Tantric love: feeling vs emotion: golden rules to make love easy*. London: O-Books.

Richardson, D. (2011). *Slow sex*. London: O-Books.

Rosenberg, M. (2003). *Non-violent communication: A language of life*. Encinitas, CA: Puddledancer Press.

Rowett, L. (2018). 'Sex, intimacy, and relationship coaching'. Available at: https://lucyrowett.com/sex-intimacy-relationship-coaching/?r_done=1

Ruiz, D. M. (1997). *The four agreements*. San Rafael, CA: Amber-Allen Publishing.

Tolle, E. (2006). *The power of now*. London: Penguin.

Valentine-Chase, M. (2020). 'Sex coaching London'. Available at: https://www.sexcoaching.london/about-sex-coaching

Wilson, C. (2017). *The work and life of David Grove*. Leicester: Troubadour Publishing.

Part 3

The SGT model

Introduction to Part 3

Part 3 of this book will explore Willem Poppeliers' psychosexual[1] stages in some depth before giving an idea of how these may be applied, firstly in the SGT work itself and then in psychotherapy generally. The section will conclude with a detailed account of how the work is practised, particularly in terms of the boundaries and regulation, which, as I've indicated in the last chapter, are important when working with sexual issues at depth.

Poppeliers' SGT model envisages psychosexual development as a life-long process, which it divides into eight stages. As with most stage theories, for example Erikson's psychosocial stages (Erikson, 1963), the chronological age assigned to each stage is flexible and the resolution of each stage doesn't prevent the individual from coming up against the issues which are relevant to the next. This will become clearer as I describe each stage in a bit more detail. In my exploration of each of the stages, I will be describing both the content, what is happening to the human being at each stage, and what Willem Poppeliers refers to as the 'parental function', or what the optimal response of a parent to their developing son or daughter is at each stage.

The diagram below gives an overview of psychosexual energetic development. The rise of the curve is deliberate, illustrating the increase of available (sexual) energy from childhood to early adulthood, the steady state of that energy during adulthood and middle age and the decrease as we begin to age. I will refer to the labels as I describe each stage.

As you can see from Figure 1.1, Willem Poppeliers divides psychosexual development into eight stages. Revelation begins at about four years old and is so called because it is the age when children not only become aware of their genitals but also have an impulse to share this awareness with those around them. Poppeliers places the next stage, Puberty, at around 14, later perhaps than is physiologically evident, but in doing this he is separating the physiological changes from the psychological adjustment to those changes. Likewise, the next stage, Adolescence, is placed at the age of 24, by which time the physiological changes to the body and the young adult's adjustment to them is complete.

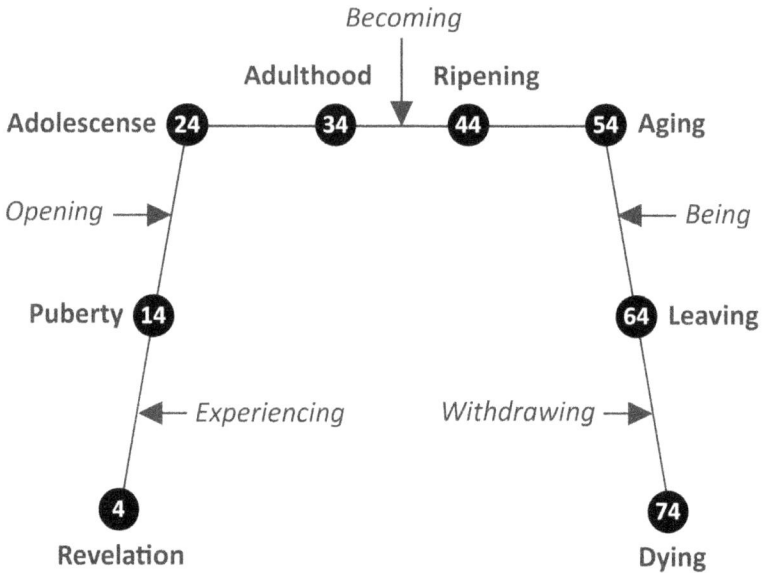

Figure 1.1 The curve of psychosexual development

Adulthood, the next stage, is again later in Poppeliers' system than current usage of that word might suggest. The reasons for this are explored in Chapter 7 and Chapter 8. The stage of Ripening, at age 44, should be self-explanatory as is the Aging stage at 54, although some people who are going through these stages may be in denial about this. All of these three stages, which form the top line of the diagram, are concerned with the harmonisation or balancing of masculinity and femininity, both internally and externally.

The Leaving stage, at 64, is as much about the process of withdrawal as about what we are leaving behind for future generations. At this, and at the previous stage, we may well be having to deal with the loss of one or both of our parents as well as the independence of our children and the effect of these is explored in Chapter 10 and Chapter 11. In locating the Dying stage at 74, Poppeliers is aware of the considerable variation in mortality, which is as much dependent on class and wealth as anything else, as is becoming increasingly apparent. One of the unique features of Sexual Grounding Therapy (SGT), as I explore in Chapter 12, is that it looks forward as well as backwards (as is the case with most psychotherapeutic models). Looking forward towards one's own death, psychosexually, is also a unique feature of SGT (see Chapter 11).

Note

1   In *Sexual Grounding Therapy*, Poppeliers uses the term 'genital-relational' rather than 'psychosexual' to describe these stages (Poppeliers & Broesterhuizen, 2007, p. 3). I

can understand this preference, particularly as a response to the *exclusion* of genitals from most of the bodywork which was being practiced at the time he developed SGT, but I have chosen the word 'psychosexual'. I have done this partly because it builds a bridge between the familiar concept in other theories and the new ideas of SGT and partly because I want to emphasise that psychosexual development happens in all human beings, however well or badly their sexuality is supported by their parents and by society in general. What SGT brings to the therapeutic world is its emphasis on the importance of parental relationships that include sexuality, embodied in both children's and parents' genitals.

References

Erikson, E. (1963). *Childhood and society*. New York: W. W. Norton & Co.

Poppeliers, W., & Broesterhuizen, M. (2007). *Sexual grounding therapy*. Breda: Protocol Media Productions.

Chapter 5

Revelation – the Oedipal stage

As I've already mentioned, Freud's work on childhood sexuality was both pioneering and controversial. Up until that time the way children were seen was contradictory. They were born, according to the church, in a state of original sin from which baptism freed them, but the resulting innocence excluded their sexuality. However, in acknowledging childhood sexual feelings and impulses, Freud seems to have viewed these through an adult lens. The Oedipal stage of psychosexual development, according to Freud, involves the young boy of 4–6 years old having the desire to have sex with his mother and kill his father. In this, Freud makes use of the original Oedipus myth, which was used by Sophocles in *Oedipus Rex*, with which Freud, as a classical scholar, would have been familiar. What Freud seems to have conveniently forgotten is that, in the play, Oedipus was a young man strong enough and skilled enough in arms to be realistically, but unknowingly, able to kill his father, wise enough to solve the riddle of the Sphinx and mature enough to father two children, again unknowingly, with Jocasta his mother. Not a young boy between 4 and 6 then!

But Freud was onto something. Children, usually at about the age of 4, *do* become interested in their own and others' genitals, especially their parents', and often have a strong desire for physical contact with their parents that includes their genitals, but is not, from the child's perspective, sexual. Many critiques of Freud's Oedipal theories centre on the lack of cross-cultural evidence and most leave the sex out or at least downplay it. Two of Freud's most prominent followers, Jung and Adler, cited Freud's overemphasis on childhood sexuality as part of their reason for breaking with the Freudian mainstream and Freud himself, according to Reich, de-emphasised the sexual aetiology of neurosis when he started to talk in terms of a 'death instinct' in the 1920s (see Reich, 1973).

Willem Poppeliers, on the other hand, leaves the sex in but looks at it from a 4–6-year-old's perspective. At this age, children not only become aware of the excitement in their own genitals, which can certainly happen before this age, but also, crucially at this age, become interested in, and curious about, similarity and difference at a genital level. According to Sexual Grounding theory, there is also an impulse to share this interest.

In Freud's version, the Oedipus complex, the term he applies to the triangular relationship at this stage, is resolved by the boy giving up his desire to have sex with his mother under threat of castration by his more powerful father, whom he internalises in the form of a punishing superego. This part of the psyche, according to Freud, has the function of controlling the unruly impulses of the id and is necessary for the establishment and maintenance of a civilised society (see Freud, 2010). Thus, although he was quite scathing about superstition and religion (see Freud, 1991), Freud seems to be endorsing a concept that is very much like original sin.

Freud's version of the Oedipus complex and its resolution for girls is equally if not more problematic. According to Freud, the girl has a similar sexual impulse towards her father as the boy has towards his mother, but, since she can see that she doesn't have a penis, she believes she has already been castrated. Two processes result from this. First, she develops penis envy, believing her mother to be an inferior being because she doesn't have one, which is resolved, when she is able to internalise her mother as her superego into a desire for a baby. Second, she moves the centre of her sexual excitement from the 'infantile' clitoris to the more adult vagina.

In his SGT model, Willem Poppeliers sees nothing that needs resolving, although he does recognise that, given the state of humanity's relationship with its own sexuality in most cultures in the world, it can easily seem that way. In this way, he is much more humanistic and much less deterministic than Freud and his followers. In Poppeliers' vision of the Oedipal stage of development, no one has to give anything up and the effect on the developing child is sex positive.

A well-adjusted man has no reason to have feelings of rivalry towards his son just because that son is curious about his mother's body and desires an innocent genital contact with her (in Sexual Grounding theory, the word 'genital' is used, especially at the Revelation stage, in this case to refer to contact involving the genitals, which, to the child at this age, are an exciting part of the body but not *sexual* in the adult sense). Instead, well-adjusted parents should both be able to recognise that the boy is seeking a positive response to a new, conscious and physical aspect of himself that he is in the process of discovering, and it is important that both parents respond positively to this.

The use of the term 'well-adjusted' in the above paragraph leads to an important concept in the Sexual Grounding model, which is that of the 'ideal parent'. This is nothing to do with perfection, which, as Winnicott observes, 'belongs to machines', but is equivalent to his idea of the 'good enough' parent (Winnicott, 1965, p. 87). When I'm talking about what children need from parents at the psychosexual stages I'm describing, I'm assuming the existence of an ideal parent who can satisfy this need. How this works therapeutically for clients who, by definition, won't have experienced ideal parenting will be discussed later. What's important here is Poppeliers' belief that the conflicts and repressions, which Freud describes in his Oedipal theory, are not an inevitable consequence of being human, although they are perhaps a *result* of the 'civilisation' which Freud himself defended in *Civilisation and its Discontents* (Freud, 2010).

The reason that Willem Poppeliers refers to the Oedipal stage as 'Revelation' is that, for both boys and girls, their development as sexual beings is being revealed, not only to themselves, but also to their parents. The optimal response from both parents is something he calls 'genital mirroring' (see my previous comment on the use of the word 'genital' at the Revelation stage) (Poppeliers & Broesterhuizen, 2007).

This is similar, as I've already mentioned, to Winnicott's idea of 'mirroring' at a much earlier stage of development. In Winnicott's version, the infant needs a positive response from his/her primary carer to their, usually nonverbal, communications, e.g., smiles and eye contact. What is mirrored in this case is the child's existence or being. The positive message that the infant unconsciously internalises is 'It's ok – more than ok – to be me and when I'm me I can expect a positive response from the world'. Winnicott is clear, though, that this expectation holds only for the early part of infancy – what he calls the omnipotent stage. He also believes that the function of the parent is also to 'fail' the child, in other words to not be perfect, within a loving relationship, which also allows the infant to feel 'held' (Winnicott, 1960).

At the Revelation stage, according to Poppeliers, the child also needs mirroring, a welcoming response to him/her as a *genital* being. The message here is something like 'It's more than ok to be a little boy/little girl with a penis/vulva, which is a beautiful part of your body. You're (usually) like one of us and different from the other'. One thing that's really helpful in being able to mirror a child of this age is the ability to access, or be aware of, that young part of oneself as a parent, in all its playfulness, innocence and excitement. Of course, this would require an optimal experience of this psychosexual stage in the parent's own life, which highlights Poppeliers' belief that psychosexual problems, which develop as a result of not being appropriately genitally mirrored, are trans-generational. Here again, the similarity with Winnicott's view on good enough mothering is striking (he believed that, in order to be a good enough mother, a woman needed to have been well enough mothered herself).

Children, at this stage of development, often spontaneously show off their genitals both to each other and particularly to their parents. This is when they need to be positively mirrored in the way I've suggested. Of course, it's not always appropriate, or even safe, for them to do this (i.e., show off their genitals), and it is the responsibility of parents to teach them this. There is clearly some internalising of regulation going on here, as I've mentioned elsewhere in this book, but it's important to distinguish between what is essentially a kindly protective regulation (in the same way as we need to teach children about crossing the road, etc.) and the punishment/shaming, which often occurs when we as adults are embarrassed by our children's lack of inhibition. As with any other impulses, which are essentially about meeting their needs, the important message that children need to internalise is that, whilst it isn't always possible or appropriate for their need to be met (in this case to be affirmed as a genital being), there's nothing wrong with the impulse itself or with them for having it.

In looking forward to Poppeliers' next stage of psychosexual development, it is important to note that he doesn't follow Freud's idea of a latency period, arguing instead that the developing child continues to need mirroring, which, during this period, needs to evolve from genital mirroring towards sexual mirroring, as well as to have their excitement, curiosity and innocence recognised, supported and regulated in the way I have described above.

References

Freud, S. (1991). *The future of an illusion*. London: Penguin.

Freud, S. (2010). *Civilisation and its discontents*. New York: W. W. Norton & Co.

Poppeliers, W., & Broesterhuizen, M. (2007). *Sexual grounding therapy*. Breda: Protocol Media Productions.

Reich, W. (1973). *The function of the orgasm*. New York: Noonday Press.

Winnicott, D. W. (1960). 'The theory of the parent-infant relationship'. *Journal of Psychoanalysis*, 41, 585–595.

Winnicott, D. W. (1965). *The maturational process and the facilitating environment*. Madison, CT: International Universities Press.

Chapter 6

Puberty and adolescence

It is fairly common in our culture for parents to sympathise with each other when their children are approaching, or in the process of, Puberty. This process, which involves growing independence from parents, developing an individual identity, especially a sexual identity, along with physiological change and growth, can be challenging for both parents and young people. One way of handling this is for parents to 'batten down the hatches' and try to establish some more or less effective boundaries to contain the worst of the teenage rebellion and pray for the arrival of some kind of maturity. I think most of us who've been parents would like to do (or have done) more than that. Sexual Grounding Therapy (SGT), regrettably, doesn't have any magic bullets that might enable parents to come through this difficult period completely unscathed. However, as is its principle throughout the model, by putting the child at the centre and focusing on what that child needs, some useful guidelines may emerge. More importantly, the therapy itself can enable adult clients to recognise what they may have needed at this stage of their lives and didn't get and to recoup this deficit. If, having had this therapeutic experience, they find themselves in the position of being a parent (or grandparent) of a young person going through this stage, they will certainly be in a better position to know what's needed.

Like young children at the Revelation stage, teenagers are full of excitement, curiosity and innocence, especially about their own and others' developing sexuality. These three concepts, together with the idea of regulation, which at the early stages of psychosexual development comes mostly from parents, are crucial to the way SGT regards all of the stages of psychosexual development. So, one of the most important things needed at this stage is for the qualities of excitement, curiosity and innocence, which present themselves in many different forms at this stage, to be recognised and supported by parents and educators within a regulatory framework. Recognising the first two is not so difficult for many adults these days, but recognising the innocence of teenagers who seem to be hell bent on making adults' lives difficult presents our culture with serious problems, and regulating these three qualities is seen as an inevitable conflict, just as the Oedipal conflict was seen as inevitable by Freud. Similarly, regulation, rather than repression or control, seems to be difficult to achieve.

Once again, adults who have probably not had a good experience of Puberty and Adolescence themselves can find it difficult to regulate and mirror their children's experience going through this stage. The mirroring required here is similar but different to and more complicated than that required at the Revelation stage. Parents were all teenagers once, and being able to remember and reconnect with that experience means that the way they relate to their teenage children will reflect that experience and therefore be more empathic. This is difficult because teenagers are resistant to acknowledging that their parents were ever young and especially that they may have been interested in sex when they were young or indeed at any age!

The physiological changes that take place during this period are profoundly challenging, both to the young people themselves and to their parents. As bodies and mental/emotional processes change, identity, as Erikson (1963) observes, and self-image become important. One thing that teenagers really need to know is that they are attractive and therefore acceptable to their peers and perhaps especially to the gender(s) to whom they themselves are attracted. This is where mirroring becomes important, but because the teenagers, who are in the process of becoming a man or a woman, are much more sophisticated than they were at age 5 or 6, the mirroring needs to be much more subtle.

Unlike children at the Revelation stage, teenagers *are* aware of adult sexuality, both in themselves and in the world around them, which includes their parents. They are unlikely to display their genitals to anybody let alone their parents; instead, it is the secondary sexual characteristics in both boys and girls that need to be noticed and yet at the same time not noticed by their parents. The important message they need to hear at this stage is something like, 'I'm noticing that you're becoming an attractive young man/woman and I'm proud of you, but I'm not going to make a big deal out of it'.

The subtlety of this recognition can be problematic in a number of different ways. Parents might, if they equate innocence with an absence or unawareness of sexuality for instance, mourn the loss of that innocence when their children become more obviously sexual beings. In some cases, parents might want to keep their children young, not just limiting the information they have about sex, which is well-nigh impossible in this day and age, but also restricting their opportunities to form sexual relationships. Both of these are less than ideal, but the way in which they, as parents, respond to their children's emerging sexuality, verbally and non-verbally, is equally if not more important.

Responding to this transition from child to adult could be seen as walking a tightrope or, perhaps more usefully, as demanding a good sense of balance from parents. In becoming young men and women, teenagers are also becoming sexually attractive and parents are not immune from this. As Searles puts it:

To me it makes sense that the more a woman loves her husband, the more she will love, similarly, the lad who is, to at least a considerable degree, the younger edition of the man she loved enough to marry.

(Searles, 2018, p. 296)

However, the crucial phrase in this sentence is 'the more a woman loves her husband' and Searles, who is talking about his own wife and son here, is assuming a well-adjusted loving couple – ideal parents as SGT theory would see it.

Other less than ideal parents may respond differently. They can, for example, respond to their teenagers' need for recognition of their developing sexuality as an invitation into an adult relationship. This *can* in some cases, especially with fathers and daughters, lead to actual sexual abuse, but it can also play out in more subtle ways, particularly when the relationship between the parents is going through a difficult phase. Female clients in my practice have reported a sexual undertone to their relationship with their father at this stage sometimes, but not always, with inappropriate comments on their developing body. Whether it's physical or emotional, this 'special' relationship with their father can often exclude or denigrate their mother.

This is confusing to the adolescent girl because she *wants* to be special to her father, but she knows that physiologically she's in the process of turning into a woman like her mother, who is the one being excluded and put down. This can not only cut her off from her mother, the parent who is best placed to support her in her journey towards womanhood, but can also lead to her being internally conflicted about her own identity as a woman – a kind of auto-misogyny. There can be a sense of alienation from her own body, the changes in which seem to be generating uncomfortable interest from her father and other men. This resistance to her own femininity, could, in extreme cases, be a contributory factor to the kind of gender dysmorphia that is becoming prevalent currently. It is beyond the scope of this book to do more than raise this as a speculation, but this dynamic is certainly not what a teenage girl needs.

With boys/young men and their mothers, it's usually different, with the inappropriate closeness being more at a feeling level. However, it's still sexual in a broad sense and is sometimes accompanied by the exclusion or denigration of the boy's father. To be fair, fathers often exclude themselves, perhaps because of their own experiences at this stage of development, and can end up being either physically or emotionally absent.

The boy certainly needs his growth into manhood to be welcomed and recognised by his mother, but he doesn't need the emotional closeness, which is often tinged with the disappointment his mother experiences in her relationship with his father. Nick Duffell and Helena Løvendal refer to this kind of inappropriate closeness in *Sex, Love and the Dangers of Intimacy* as 'heart rape' (Duffell & Løvendal, 2006). Although this may sound over-dramatic, there is no doubt that men who have had this kind of invasive relationship with their mothers can find it difficult to emotionally connect with their partners later in life. This mother/son dynamic is brilliantly characterised in D. H. Lawrence's autobiographical novel, *Sons and Lovers* (Lawrence, 1981), which also gives a vivid account of the effects of this distorted type of relationship on future adult relationships. In the novel, it is only after the death of his mother that the protagonist Paul Morel finally experiences a liberation, which enables him to realise that neither of the two relationships he has had so far have been particularly healthy, together with some sort of rapprochement with his father.

The other way in which fathers can respond to their daughters' emerging sexuality is with fear, not only of what's happening to their 'little girl', but also of their own response to it. In some cases, this can lead to attempts to control the daughter in terms of her dress, social activities, etc., but often the father's fear of his own sexual response to his daughter's sexual development leads to withdrawal or rejection, especially as far as physical affection is concerned. Suddenly the cuddles and hugs stop and the girl is left feeling abandoned and unsupported without knowing what she's done wrong.

In the Sexual Grounding model, what the girl who is becoming a young woman really needs from her father is a recognition of her emerging sexuality at a feeling or heart level, rather than at a sexual or genital level. He appreciates and is proud of her beauty but without the need to possess her sexually himself. To quote Searles (2018) again:

> If a little girl cannot feel herself able to win the heart of her father, her own father who has known her so well and for so long, and who is tied to her by mutual blood-ties, I reasoned, then how can the young woman who comes later have any deep confidence in the power of her womanliness?
>
> (p. 296)

Willem Poppeliers would go beyond Searles and suggest that, in meeting his daughter's need as described above, a father can enable her to develop a deep and intimate trust of men.

With mothers and sons, the equivalent is that mothers are not only less physical when their sons start to become young men but also repress all interest in what is happening for their sons sexually, both in terms of the boys' physical and emotional development and of their first ventures into the world of sexual relationships. It's as if the changes in their sons' bodies and in their emotional worlds are just not happening. Normal teenage masturbation is ignored and therefore becomes a dirty secret to be ashamed of. The existence, or not, of girlfriends/boyfriends is a matter of indifference.

This distancing can sometimes be associated with criticism along the lines of 'You're just as bad as your father', from which the boy learns that there is something wrong with his masculinity. It's clearly not ok to be like his father, but he clearly *is* like his father, both genetically and genitally. This is exacerbated in families where the father, sometimes for understandable reasons, gets treated like one of the children rather than a husband.

Of course, all teenagers have two parents, whether they live with them or not, and their relationship with their parent of the same sex is equally crucial. Although teenagers may seem oblivious to their parents and self-absorbed, they are actually observing their parents closely and learning about how to be a man or a woman, even though this is sometimes seen in terms of, 'I never want to be like him/her'. As I said earlier, there is a lot of excitement, curiosity and re innocence associated with this period of psychosexual development and the role of parents is to support this, whilst at the same time also supporting their teenage children in becoming self-regulating.

Much is written about the issue of 'consent' at the moment, rightly so, and parents have a critical role here during their children's teenage years. SGT would see this as an issue of regulation. A teenage girl needs to know that it's more than ok to say 'no' to a sexual activity if it doesn't feel right to her, but also that it's more than ok for her to say 'yes' if it does feel right. Learning this verbally, either at school or from their parents is better than nothing, but it doesn't really get taken in on an unconscious, body level. Also, for what seem to be understandable reasons, the emphasis in Sex and Relationship Education and in advice from parents is more on the 'no' than the 'yes'. Fear and control are once more in evidence. In order to fully understand consent, according to the SGT model, the girl needs to experience her mother as a sexual woman who can and does say 'yes' to sex and who is also confident enough to say 'no' as well.

The question is: how does a daughter get to know/experience her mother like this? Much is written about mother/daughter relationships during Adolescence, and Kim McCabe's excellent programme gives much needed support to both daughters and mothers in the process of the latter supporting their daughters in their transition into womanhood (McCabe, 2018). The SGT model takes a similar but more therapeutic perspective. An ideal mother will be comfortable with her own sexuality and impulses. These are actually what she's saying 'yes' or 'no' to, as well as to the man or woman with whom she may or may not want to have sex, and what she can usefully teach her daughter about. She will express this both in her demeanour and in the way she responds to her daughter's curiosity and excitement about sex. If she can contact the teenager in herself whilst at the same time being in touch with herself as a mature, self-regulated woman, she will be able to mirror her daughter's excitement and curiosity without the anxiety, which can so often lead to control and prohibition.

Young people are very sensitive to these 'vibes' in the adults around them and will clam up if they experience an incongruity between what adults are saying and how they're feeling on the inside. As I write this, I'm aware that it can sound as if Willem Poppeliers is expecting and encouraging young people to expect an awful lot from parents: the kind of perfection I was describing earlier in my discussion of Winnicott (1965), which, as he says, belongs to machines (p. 87). Actually, young people are very tolerant of the human frailty in the adults around them. Once again, it's not so much about being perfect as being 'good enough', and this involves parents acknowledging their own vulnerability and experience. The alternative is presenting the false picture of either being totally laid back about sex and having found it all perfectly straightforward or of never having had sex or sexual desires other than in marriage for the purposes of procreation. Being 'good enough' is also about moving in the right direction (i.e., towards a positive view and experience of sex) and acknowledging that, if you haven't got there yet, that's your problem and your work in progress.

Although the issue of *their own* consent to sex can be an issue for boys and men, it is perhaps more important, in our present culture, that young men learn how to regulate themselves in relation to young women's responses to their sexual advances. In the SGT model, Willem Poppeliers would argue that this isn't *just* a matter of culture but also because men generally feel more vulnerable at a heart or feeling level, and women generally feel more vulnerable at a genital or sexual level (Poppeliers & Broesterhuizen, 2007, p. 41). In this he is influenced by the tantric idea of the human body as an electromagnet[1] with men having their plus pole in their genitals and their minus pole in their heart and women being the other way around (see Richardson, 2003), and, like Diana Richardson, he also believes that physical form, in terms of male and female bodies, is important in this respect. Essentially, the belief that SGT shares with Tantra is that each sex gives out energetically from their plus pole and receives in their minus pole and that this is reflected in the physical form of men and women.

The implication of this is that, for young men, it is more of an issue to consent (commit) to emotional intimacy than it is to consent to sex, and there's plenty of, admittedly anecdotal, evidence to support this. I need to be clear that I'm not saying that this gender difference between where plus and minus poles are located constitutes a 'get out of jail free card' for men as far as commitment is concerned any more than I'm saying that young women are incapable of managing consent or initiation in sex. I'm much more interested in what young people in our current culture need from parents during their teenage years in order to develop and maintain respectful and fulfilling sexual relationships. For each gender, to have parental support in their minus pole enhances this possibility. I have already described how this works for girls and their mothers and will illustrate what boys need from their fathers below.

What support do boys need in learning about consent? As with girls, they can learn the *information* either from their parents or at school, but the additional danger here is that this becomes internalised as some kind of 'rule', control rather than (self) regulation, which then has the effect of strengthening the impulse – feeding it by making it more exciting. This is similar to what I observed about sex and Christianity in Chapter 1. Confused young men have been known to resort to using their smartphones to record a young woman's consent in order to avoid being accused of non-consensual acts.

A more effective strategy is for parents, especially fathers, to recognise their sons' innocence, support their curiosity and excitement and teach them, mostly by example, how to regulate these. If a boy can experience his father as a loving, responsive man (by implication, a man who is in touch with his heart), both in relation to his mother and to himself, a man who is brave enough to take the initiative sexually but also sensitive and confident enough to accept a 'no' without feeling diminished, he will then have a model of consent in action, which he can internalise.

As with mothers and daughters, it is unlikely that boys will actually witness this kind of interaction (i.e., the initiation of sex) between their parents, but the modelling will be present in the overall 'climate' of their parents' relationship and will also be present in fathers' responses to their questions about sex and relationships.

What emerges from the above discussion about consent is that, as far as Sexual Grounding is concerned, young people need different things from each parent. Curiously, support at a genital or sexual level comes from the mother for both sons and daughters, and support at a heart level comes from the father. Sadly, as has been observed by therapists such as Terry Real (2002), although women have begun to empower themselves sexually, most men remain unavailable at a heart level, which makes this much needed support for their offspring a rare commodity.

At the Revelation stage, it is certainly true that social context has an influence on the developing child, but, other than via kindergarten teachers and grandparents, etc., this influence is mostly mediated by their parents. At the stage of Puberty and Adolescence, it is the young people themselves who are directly exposed to their social context, of which social media and the internet are probably the most influential.

As I've already commented, we live in an era where there is more information about sex than there has ever been and fewer taboos on how sex can be discussed, experienced and practised. Willem Poppeliers believes that today's society is over-excited by sex and sees the proliferation of pornography and the use of sex to support consumer culture as examples of this. For young people this is particularly difficult because they are at the stage of exploring themselves as sexual beings in relation to their peers for the first time and full of curiosity and excitement. When the acknowledgement of their emerging sexuality is absent in the home, they are strongly attracted to other sources of information and experience. Acutely self-conscious about the physical changes in their bodies and without much affirmation of their self-image as a young man or woman, young people can come to believe that they need to look and behave like the actors they see on the screen, both in the popular media and in the porn industry in order to be considered attractive.

In *Sex in Class*, a controversial 2015 documentary about sex education in British schools directed by Lisa Poulter, presenter Goedele Liekens seriously challenged these adolescent beliefs, and this was on the whole well received by the young people themselves. She was met with much more resistance by the parents whom she tried to involve in their children's sex education. The documentary met with a mixed response at the time and, as far as I'm aware, hasn't been followed up in British schools (there certainly isn't, as she proposed, a GCSE in sex and relationships!) although Sex and Relationship Education has now become a compulsory part of the curriculum in all schools. From an SGT perspective, the difficulty with Sex and Relationship Education in schools is that there are hardly any people like Goedele Liekens, who could be seen as an ideal parent figure, available to teach the subject.

Willem Poppeliers identifies two other problems with pornography. The first is that, by definition, it privileges the visual stimulus over all other senses, which can result in difficulty when encountering the real, flawed human being, who doesn't have a perfect vulva with a total absence of pubic hair or a gigantic penis that is permanently erect, who is much more likely to be their actual partner. Whilst the neurological evidence is inconclusive, demonstrating a correlation rather than a causal connection (Kühn & Gallinat, 2014), it has been suggested that an excess of visual stimuli will result in a desensitisation of other more tactile or olfactory stimuli. Certainly, the increasing frequency of erectile dysfunction in young men may well be connected to this phenomenon. The second problem Poppeliers identifies is that the vast majority of depictions of sexual acts in por-nography involve no feeling or emotional contact between the participants. As he puts it: 'The goal is to cause excitement, free of intimacy. The image young people acquire of sexuality diminishes into an egotistical need for discharge' (Poppeliers & Broesterhuizen, 2007, p. 39).

Curiously, Freud's 'fluid mechanics' model of libido based on charge and discharge (cathexis and catharsis) would appear to support this version of sexual satisfaction.

In contrast, the lived experience of sexuality as an expression of love and respect strongly associated with shared feelings and intimacy, whilst less exciting, promises fulfilment and lasting relationships. It is easy to forget that Adolescence is a time of emotional exploration and experimentation, not to mention idealism and sexual discovery, when working with adolescents and contemplating Adolescence's dangers and difficulties. Willem Poppeliers is certainly not endorsing a return to Puritanism in the upbringing of adolescents, but he is keen to see the link strengthened between genital activity and feeling/intimacy.

Although young people have probably always seen themselves as different from the adults around them, the phenomenon of the 'teenager' is a fairly recent development in human history and owes as much to the advertising and marketing industries as it does to the existence of teenagers as a distinct social group. The Google dictionary, which also has a facility for tracing the fre-quency with which a word is mentioned over time, records that the word 'teenager' was scarcely used at all before 1950. Different fashions, genres of music and modes of behaviour serve the purpose of enabling young people to feel confirmed in their identity (Erikson, 1963), but this is fuelled only partly by this need and is ruthlessly exploited as a source of revenue by the media, fashion and music industries.

There are advantages to the emergence of a distinct teenage category, since it gives recognition and identity to this age group and legitimises their feeling of being different. The downside is that it cuts them off from the adults who could support their transition and also cuts the adults off, not just from the young people in their lives, but also from the younger more adventurous part of themselves, which would enable them, as I've said, to mirror their teenage off-spring's excitement, curiosity and innocence, albeit from a regulated position. The other thing that's really important about maintaining contact between adults and teenagers is that the transition I referred to above is anything but linear. Teenagers will fluctuate wildly between being 'super adult' one minute and dependent 5-year-olds the next. Telling them to 'act their age' or abandoning them, perhaps in revenge for feeling abandoned *by* them or perhaps just to avoid the stress of dealing with the Jekyll and Hyde-like characters they seem to have become, is counterproductive to say the least.

As I've already remarked, there is no perfect way to bring up a teenager or a child of any age, and this is certainly not what Willem Poppeliers is talking about in his Sexual Grounding model. A more sex-positive context, by which I mean that parents and influential adults in teenagers' lives are doing their best to live their own sexuality in a fulfilling and loving context whilst at the same time supporting their offspring in learning to do the same, is much more what's needed for both adults and teenagers alike. The important transition that is happening during this period is from external regulation of the excitement, curiosity and innocence, which are all components of intimate relationships, to self-regulation, which is necessary for the move into adulthood that comes with the next psychosexual stage.

Note

1 The idea of the body literally generating a magnetic field is accepted in many of the alternative healing professions, but a discussion of this is beyond the scope of this book. In the present context, the idea of plus and minus poles can be regarded as metaphorical.

References

Duffell, N., & Løvendal, H. (2006). *Sex, love and the dangers of intimacy.* London: Harper Collins.

Erikson, E. (1963). *Childhood and society.* New York: W. W. Norton & Co.

Kühn, S., & Gallinat, J. (2014). 'Brain structure and functional connectivity associated with pornography consumption'. *JAMA Psychiatry*, 71(7), 827–834.

Lawrence, D. H. (1981). *Sons and lovers.* London: Penguin.

McCabe, K. (2018). *From daughter to woman.* London: Robinson.

Poppeliers, W., & Broesterhuizen, M. (2007). *Sexual grounding therapy*. Breda: Protocol Media Productions.

Poulter, L. (Director). (2015). *Sex in class*. Film. London: Ricochet.

Real, T. (2002). *How can I get through to you?* New York: Simon & Schuster.

Richardson, D. (2003). *The heart of tantric sex*. London: O-Books.

Searles, H. (2018). *Collected papers on schizophrenia and related subjects*. London: Routledge.

Winnicott, D. W. (1965). *The maturational process and the facilitating environment*. Madison, CT: International Universities Press.

Chapter 7

Adolescence to adulthood

Whilst young people are regarded as adults financially and politically from the age of 18, and sexually adult at 16, the stage of Adulthood in Sexual Grounding Therapy (SGT) begins at around the age of 24, when Adolescence ends. At around this age – sometimes later these days – the experimentation with sexual identity, which in SGT means how you feel inside about yourself as a sexual being rather than what gender pronouns you prefer or who you direct your sexual desires towards, has ideally enabled the young man or woman to know themselves sexually. From this position they are able to become interested in establishing a relationship whose purpose is simply to *be* a relationship rather than to confirm the identity of one or both participants. This, of course, is the theory. In reality, many relationships do retain some of the latter goal and this, almost inevitably, according to Nick Duffell and Helena Løvendal leads to problems in the relationship when the partners are unable and/or unwilling to do this for each other (Duffell & Løvendal, 2005). Duffell and Løvendal see this as an opportunity for the relationship to grow and develop rather than as a problem which needs to be solved.

The projection of one or both of one's parents onto one's partner is well-known in couples' therapy and is the foundation of Imago Therapy (Hendrix, 2005). In SGT, this is known as a 'triadic relationship', with the projected parent(s) becoming the 'third thing' in the relationship and getting in the way of the intimacy. We avoid meeting our real partner in a 'dyadic relationship', which SGT would see as ideal or Sexually Grounded. I've highlighted the expression 'dyadic relationship' because it has a particular meaning in SGT, that is to say a relationship where there is no projection on either side. I can best illustrate this by offering the reader an experiential dyadic exercise:

> To do this exercise you will need a partner, not necessarily a sexual partner but someone you feel physically comfortable with. Find a position where you're separate from each other but close enough to hold hands. Hold your partner's hand, and each of you focus your awareness in the following manner:

1   I feel *your hand and* you feel *my hand*.
2   *I feel your hand*, which is feeling my hand *and you feel my hand*, which is feeling your hand.
3   *I feel your hand feeling my hand*, feeling our hands *and you feel my hand feeling your hand* feeling our hands.
4   *I feel our hands* feeling each other's feeling of our hands *and you feel our hands* feeling each other's feeling of our hands.

The emphases indicate the focus of awareness and, although at one level the instructions for this exercise can read like a passage from R. D. Laing's 'Knots' (Laing, 1970), experienced physically rather than linguistically, they demonstrate the core contact, which is only possible in a dyadic relationship.

Whatever the state of both partners' security in their identities and however imperfect they are, relationships do tend to become more permanent at around this age, whether or not the couples choose to get married or form a civil partnership. According to SGT, this is where parents, and especially parents-in-law, become important, as Willem Poppeliers would put it, as the sexual sources of one's potential life partner.

As I've said, although most therapies consider the influence of parents at this stage of life to be fairly unimportant except as far as the unresolved childhood issues are concerned, SGT considers both parents and parents-in-law as essential in supporting what is often a fragile relationship in its early stages. It is significant that it is the *relationship* rather than the individual son or daughter that needs supporting at this stage. Of course, all parents will, hopefully, feel a bond with their own son or daughter, but at this stage, supporting *them*, rather than the relationship is often more a matter of possessiveness and can be damaging (to the relationship). Curiously, this dynamic is very similar to that advocated by many schools of couples' therapy, i.e., seeing the relationship as the client rather than either of the individuals. Perhaps couples' therapists occupy the space left by the lack of supportive relationships with parents and parents-in-law?

As in the teenage years, support can be offered on a practical basis with information/advice and listening, but the most important thing is the example that is being set. Being able to see your parents-in-law as your partner's sexual sources is also a two-way process. This involves the young adult acknowledging that his/her parents-in-law not only made love to create their partner but also that they continued to have sex after this and are in all likelihood still doing so, even if not always with their original partner. As the parent-in-law, it is important to be visible as a sexual being who is capable of loving and respecting their partner and living their sexuality in a fulfilling manner, appropriate to their stage in life. This is one of the ways in which Poppeliers is taking us back to the way relationships were managed in indigenous cultures. In *The Spirit of Intimacy*, Sobonfu Somé (1997) talks about how, in the Dagra community in

West Africa, weddings are an occasion for the older members of the community to remember and renew their vows.

The above may seem to run counter to many people's experience where relationships with in-laws are, at best, tense and formal or, at worst, a stress on, rather than a support for, the couple's relationship. Although mother-in-law jokes have, I hope, disappeared from most comedians' repertoire, the way in-laws are portrayed in the media does little to enhance the reputation of in-laws as sources of support and guidance. This is perhaps because, just as in the two earlier stages, parents and parents-in-law are often less than ideal or good enough. However, they *have* experienced the challenges of being in a lasting relationship even when they are no longer together with the father or mother of their children (In my practice as a couple-worker, I used to tell couples who were thinking of splitting up that they would have a relationship at least until all of their children were 18. Since my involvement in SGT, I've modified this!). Parents and parents-in-law will have inevitably made mistakes in their own relationships, but they can make an important contribution to their off-spring's experience by acknowledging these so that they (the young people) can learn from them. Figure 7.1 gives an idea of the supportive matrix in which the young relationship can be supported.

One of the crucial elements of a lasting relationship is mutual understanding. This statement is hardly unique to SGT, but Willem Poppeliers sees this in terms of curiosity about the masculinity and femininity in both partners. In a heterosexual couple, the man needs to understand his own femininity in order to have an intimate and lasting relationship with his female partner and the opposite is true for the woman. In same-sex couples, it is equally important that both partners understand their own and each other's masculinity and

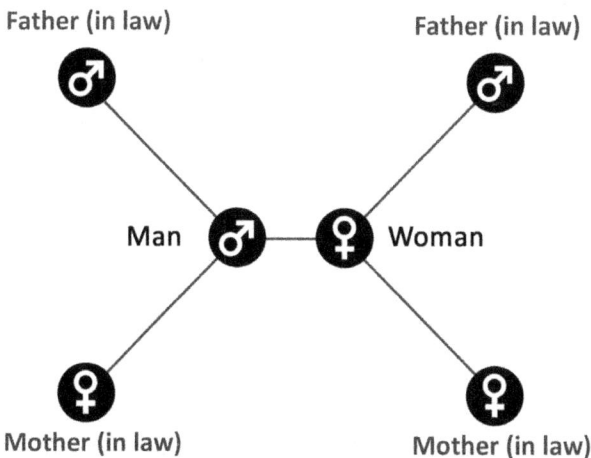

Figure 7.1 Man, woman and in-laws

femininity in order to deepen the relationship. However, whilst there is an advantage in that both partners will have similar sexual anatomy, they will also need to understand its opposite in themselves and in each other.

This is a development or maturation from the adolescent perspective where the tendency is to project one's less familiar, and sometimes therefore disowned, characteristics onto the other person in the relationship. Arguably this happens on a societal level, especially from men towards women where men project the disowned aspects of themselves – weakness, emotionality, unpredictability, lack of sexual desire, etc. – onto women, rather than owning them as part of themselves (see Horrocks, 1994).

In a lasting relationship, the issue of children is almost inevitable, one way or another. In Willem Poppeliers' formulation, sex and reproduction are inextricably linked and arguably this has its roots in the history of humankind, for most of which this has been demonstrably true. However, SGT is not a branch of the Catholic Church! The SGT position is that, when you make love, even though you may be using contraception, there is always the possibility of conceiving a baby. This is clearly true literally (there is no form of contraception that is 100% effective) as well as at a feeling or energetic level. It might be argued that this is also a possibility at the adolescent stage, so why does it become so important now? The answer is that most teenagers aren't thinking about wanting babies, except hopefully as something to avoid, when they're making love whereas for young adults the idea of starting a family is likely to be somewhere in their consciousness – see the paragraph below. Willem Poppeliers' recommendation is that 'partners try to experience sexual intercourse from their hearts in such a way that they would be able to fully accept an unplanned pregnancy' (Poppeliers & Broesterhuizen, 2007, p. 45).

In my practice as a couples' and psychosexual therapist, though, I'm quite often surprised how disconnected these processes have become, even taking account of the availability and prevalence of contraception at the present time. One or other of the couple will report, 'and then I/she got pregnant' often as a precipitating factor in some difficulty they're working on. When I ask them about contraception, they often regress to naïve (innocent) teenagers, saying things like, 'It just happened' or 'We got carried away in the moment', etc. At the very least, this signifies an unconscious wish from one or both partners for a child, but it is probably also true that the partners are not involving their hearts in the way that Willem Poppeliers recommends. As he sees it, one of the functions of the heart is to protect life. It does this literally by keeping our body alive, but it also does it, according to Sexual Grounding theory, energetically and emotionally.

Even when the couple are being careful to avoid pregnancy, it can seem that a pragmatic decision has been made, often not (fully) discussed, that now is not the right time to start a family, and there are very often understandable and sensible reasons for this. However, hearts are rarely included in the discussion, which is usually attributable to fear of the powerful feelings involved. SGT would see this as an issue of regulation where the difference between experiencing a feeling in oneself and taking it seriously in the other, and acting on it, is not embodied. In my practice as a couple therapist, I find that this is often the reason behind couples being unwilling to give space to their own, and especially each other's, feelings. They believe, perhaps unconsciously, that giving space to feelings is the same as agreeing with and maybe acting on them. Sharing the heartfelt desire for, and fear of, having children will not only bring a couple emotionally closer together but can also highlight areas where more support is needed for the relationship, which, from an SGT perspective, involves parents and parents-in-law. This is irrespective of the decision the couple arrive at as a result of this sharing.

Of course, although the above paragraphs are probably applicable to the majority of relationships, there is a significant proportion of relationships to which the principles described cannot be literally applied. Couples in same-sex relationships can and do choose to have children, but they don't have to be aware of this possibility every time they make love, as Willem Poppeliers recommends to heterosexual couples. Likewise, when/if they choose to have a baby, it's always a conscious choice requiring considerable planning. Sex and reproduction seem to be unconnected in same-sex relationships, and, at first sight, it looks as if this could create a physical, energetic distance between the couple and their offspring. However, whilst there may be a difference between this and the ideal heterosexual couple experience, it is actually comparatively rare for a heterosexual couple to 'experience sexual intercourse from their hearts in such a way that they would be able to fully accept an unplanned pregnancy' (Poppeliers & Broesterhuizen, 2007, p. 45).

Thus, as far as SGT is concerned, one difference between a heterosexual couple and a same-sex couple, in terms of conceiving children, is that the heterosexual couple needs to involve their hearts more and the same-sex couple needs to involve their genitals more. The last part of that sentence may not seem to make sense, but I will explain. In both cases, this is more of an energetic/emotional involvement than a physical one. At various of the adult stages in psychosexual development, Poppeliers talks about making love with an intention, in this case for a baby, even though, in the case of a same-sex couple or a couple who knows themselves to be infertile, this is emotional/energetic rather than literal. This idea is another of the 'spiritual implications' of the work, which I alluded to in Chapter 4, and isn't unique to SGT but also features in some tantric approaches (see Anand, 1995).

In *Sexual Grounding Therapy*, Willem Poppeliers controversially recommends that the third party, either the sperm donor or the surrogate, who he identifies as one of the child's genital sources, is involved in the upbringing of the child (Poppeliers & Broesterhuizen, 2007). The practicality of this kind of arrangement is a matter of debate, but, as with every aspect of his work, Poppeliers is putting the child at the centre and thinking about what will ideally meet their needs. I will return to the idea of the importance of biological triangles in Chapter 9.

Other couples, heterosexual or same sex, may either choose not to have children or be unable to do so due to either age or infertility. In this case SGT recommends thinking about sex, especially the giving and receiving of sexual energy, as being focused on the production of a 'third thing', which could be a mutual project or enterprise, which has an equivalent fulfilment for both partners in the relationship.

The arrival, or not, of children, invariably involves parents and parents-in-law, whether we are talking about their eagerness to become grandparents or the influence they have on the upbringing of the children. This can take many forms, including being determined not to make the same mistakes as our parents, but the influence, in whatever form it emerges, is always there. Eagerness to become grandparents could be construed as selfish, living vicariously on the part of the parents and parents-in-law. This could well be true if they are at a stagnant point either in their career, relationship or both, but Poppeliers sees this more in terms of continuing the generation line and supporting it as a function of their own age. If the parents and parents-in-law are fulfilled in themselves then they have surplus energy to support the emerging generations. Poppeliers refers to this as 'surplus value' (see Chapter 16) (W. Poppeliers, personal communication, 2020).

There are two important evolutions from Adolescence that need to happen at this stage according to the Sexual Grounding model. The first is that sex becomes more about contact with one's partner (giving and receiving) than about personal gratification. This Poppeliers equates with the quality of innocence, i.e., being open to the experience rather than goal orientated (towards orgasm). Once more it is easy to see the influence of tantric ideas here, as Diana Richardson explores in *Slow Sex* (Richardson, 2011). Although Poppeliers acknowledges that this evolution is gradual, it must be acknowledged that contactful and non-goal-oriented sex is a comparative rarity even amongst mature and well-functioning couples.

The other evolution is the move away from being regulated from the outside by parents towards self-regulation. Essentially, this involves the acknowledgement and acceptance that actions (within the relationship) have consequences. The connection between sexual intercourse and pregnancy has already been discussed, but other influences, such as infidelity, neglect and reluctance to give or receive all have consequences for the quality and intimacy of the relationship. This is where the difference between regulation and morality/control is highlighted. It's not that any of these kinds of actions are bad or sinful and deserve punishment,[1] but rather that recognising that all of our actions within a relationship have an effect for which we are accountable is a sign of maturity. Although parents and parents-in-law are no longer responsible for the regulation itself, they can occupy an important role in encouraging the couple, mostly by example, to recognise that their actions have consequences and to encourage the cooperation between them.

Note

1 It's arguable, perhaps, that abusive and coercive behaviour is an exception to this. However, it could also be argued that it is unusual for perpetrators of this behaviour to allow themselves to be truly accountable for their behaviour and to fully acknowledge the consequences.

References

Anand, M. (1995). *The art of sexual magic*. London: Piaktus.
Duffell, N., & Løvendal, H. (2005). *Love, sex and the dangers of intimacy*. London: Harper Collins.
Hendrix, H. (2005). *Getting the love you want*. London: Pocket Books.
Horrocks, R. (1994). *Masculinity in crisis*. Basingstoke: MacMillan.
Laing, R. D. (1970). *Knots*. London: Pelican.
Poppeliers, W., & Broesterhuizen, M. (2007). *Sexual grounding therapy*. Breda: Protocol Media Productions.
Richardson, D. (2011). *Slow sex*. London: O-Books.
Somé, S. (1997). *The spirit of intimacy*. New York: William Morrow.

Chapter 8

Adulthood towards ripening

As we look at this extended model of psychosexual development, it becomes clearer how divergent the pattern is becoming, both because of the individual variation within any culture and also because of changes to that culture itself. Currently, we have more choices about relationships, careers and children than at any time in history, and this can make the discussion of stage theories like SGT seem complicated. However, the latest figures from the Office for National Statistics put the average age of first time mothers at 30.3 in the UK (ONS, 2018), which suggests that the SGT model isn't totally inaccurate in suggesting that the previous stage is the most likely to be the time when young adults will form committed relationships and decide to have children.

In discussing this next stage, it is important to bear in mind that there is considerable variation behind statistics such as these. People have a choice and it isn't part of Willem Poppeliers' mission to control peoples' choices. However, life is finite and sometimes postponing goals can lead to dealing with more than one life task simultaneously or, at least, having some catching up to do. Not impossible of course, but the consequence of choices, even when those choices seem to have been forced upon us, has to be acknowledged, particularly in a therapeutic model that works with all the stages of life up to and including death. To give an example: if, like me, you leave it relatively late to have your children, and they in turn leave it relatively late to have their children, you're not going to have the energy to be as actively involved with your grandchildren as you would have been if you'd had them earlier in your life. On the other hand, you will hopefully have acquired the wisdom to be able to support your children as parents.

The 'Adulthood towards Ripening' stage, which begins at roughly 34, represents a challenge, both in terms of the development of a relationship, which may have begun in one's twenties, and also in terms of one's own personal and professional development. The relationship can be seen as a mutual support and challenge but can also be seen as an encumbrance, a limitation on one's freedom. Children are a gift, but they also make demands, which can seem to get in the way of personal and career goals. Altogether, this is a more challenging decade than it seems.

Within a relationship, it has to be acknowledged that the relationship isn't new anymore and neither are the children who are the product of that relationship. At this stage, it is common for boredom and dissatisfaction to arise, and one partner is often blaming of and at the same time blamed by the other. Parents and parents-in-law become important again at this stage in demonstrating how it can be, either to walk away and find a new partner, or stay with the routine, settling for a comfortable but unfulfilling marriage or, ideally, exploring and working through the dissatisfaction.

Far from actually being perfect, which would make a thirty-something husband or wife feel inadequate, it is important for sons and daughters (in-law) to be aware of the difficulties their parents have experienced in their relationship, whether they were able to work through them or not and of the consequences one way or the other for the relationship in the long term. In my practice, for example, I often hear one member of the couple say that their parents had a good relationship – they never heard them arguing. Although it's certainly not great to have destructive arguments in front of your children, I always feel that these parents have let their child down in that they haven't really taught them how to go through difficulties and come out of the other side, allowing the relationship, together with each partner, to grow as a result.

One trap that Willem Poppeliers identifies at this stage of psychosexual life is what he calls the 'Genital Freedom Illusion'. It is common for partners in the relationship to grow or drift apart during this decade. It can also sometimes feel as if our partner is getting in the way of our wishes and desires, especially around sex. It is not at all uncommon for one or other partner to lose interest in sex, and, understandably perhaps, it is tempting to get interested in sexual activities designed to 'spice up' the relationship, which, whilst exciting, can create more distance between partners.

There is, at the same time, a kind of closeness that can result from one partner accepting the other's suggestion of an exciting activity, which can feel like an acceptance of the desire that the activity symbolises. For example, the need to be dominated or restrained can indicate a difficulty with naturally surrendering not so much to a partner, but to one's own sexual desires and impulses. If I have this need and my partner understands, accepts and is willing to play his/her part in this, then, on the one hand, I feel understood and accepted. On the other hand, the underlying reason for that need (i.e., that I find it difficult to surrender to my sexual impulses and desires, which much more accurately represents me or my reality in that moment) has been effectively avoided.

Does this sound judgemental or pathologising? It's understandable that it might, but the impetus of Sexual Grounding Therapy is the encouragement of curiosity, in this case in the couple relationship, rather than judgement or labelling on the one hand or blanket acceptance on the other. In other words, the curiosity deepens the relationship, whether or not it changes the way your express your sexuality with each other.

In Sexual Grounding terms, introducing any 'third element' into the relationship runs the risk of it becoming 'triadic' (see Chapter 7). The projection, in this case, is onto the activity, what it symbolises or the equipment involved. Again, this is not a question of simple morality, although it is very easy to polarise this and similar psychosexual issues as morality versus freedom. Sometimes a 'third element' can be a bridge between partners and doesn't have to be necessarily sexual – a common interest for instance. In its right place, it serves a function, but it can become dominant. There's also nothing wrong with sexual experimentation and curiosity, but this can become a problem when it is an avoidance of the *relational* curiosity, i.e., curiosity about myself and/or my partner. The pursuit of individual excitement can become a substitute for fulfilment in giving and receiving and the intrinsic excitement of being (sexually) alive.

The pursuit of (apparent) freedom, in response to what is experienced as a stuck or unfulfilling relationship, can result in either the ending of the relationship or an affair. As Ester Perel (2017) observes, an affair is often about not being able to express an aspect of oneself, especially sexually, within a committed relationship. Leaving the relationship without resolving the issue of boredom or dissatisfaction creates further problems as you almost certainly end up taking the same issue into your relationship with your new partner, although it may take some time for this to become apparent. Willem Poppeliers believes that true freedom is the result of moving in the opposite direction, i.e., *towards* your partner rather than away from them, with curiosity about yourself and about your partner. Another way of expressing this is to say that true sexual freedom is the ability to be myself sexually *within* my relationship.

Part of the Freedom Illusion is the romantic idea that there is just one person, or type of person, with whom you can create a fulfilling sexual relationship. This idea is comparatively recent even in Western culture, despite the reference to the search for one's 'other half' in Aristophanes' speech in Plato's *Symposium* (Plato, 1999) and is strange to other cultures (Somé, 1997). However, letting go of this illusion is challenging.[1] The implication of doing so is that one could have a fulfilling sexual relationship with practically anybody and since most of us, however well-adjusted we believe ourselves to be, want to feel special in our relationships, there is considerable resistance here.

Poppeliers clarifies the idea by acknowledging that there are other aspects to a sexual relationship such as shared values, aspirations and life goals, which are also important for its success and that these can be important factors in one's choice of partner. However, he is also clear that if the partners in a relationship learn to express their sexual impulses and wishes fully within their relationship and cultivate mutual understanding of these, which doesn't necessarily mean enacting all of them, the relationship will grow and flourish, leading to fulfilment but not necessarily the kind of excitement that seems to be a common pursuit.

This means that both partners need to look inside themselves at what might be preventing them expressing their impulses and desires and what concerns they may have about accepting those of their partner. Otherwise, even if the 'partner blaming' referred to earlier doesn't literally happen, there is a temptation to attribute this reluctance to the characteristics or attitude of one's partner (often these are more about projection than anything else) rather than owning it oneself. This supports the idea of moving onto another partner if things aren't working, which might sometimes need to happen, especially if that partner isn't able or willing to do the personal work/exploration involved in making the expression of their needs and desires more fulsome and the acceptance of their partner's sexuality more open.

As I re-read the above paragraphs, I find myself wondering what you, the reader, are imagining when you read phrases like 'sexual impulses and wishes' and 'impulses and desires'. My suspicion is that this could include some quite exotic sexual activities! This isn't surprising, but in a Sexual Grounding context, if we take Poppeliers' idea of sexuality being about connection and fulfilment seriously, then most of the impulses and desires will be directed towards emotional and physical connection. This is what we all long for and will give us the fulfilment we're seeking.

Clearly, ideal parenting at this and the preceding stages of development would make this process of sharing our intimate selves more straightforward, but this is rare. It involves not only going against the transgenerational family dynamics (i.e., the repression of sexual desire back through the generations) but also our culture itself, which is in many ways still quite repressive.

Poppeliers goes on to suggest that, in his version of sexual freedom, universal polarities between masculinity and femininity can be experienced. He writes:

> The man sees the woman as bearer of feminine energy; as representative of all that is female, which she shapes in her own personal manner. In turn, the woman sees [the man][2] as bearer of masculine energy; as the representative of all that is male, which he shapes in his own personal manner.
>
> (Poppeliers & Broesterhuizen, 2007, p. 52)

In this free relationship, according to Poppeliers, when a man makes love to his female partner he is, in a sense, making love to all women (to femininity personified), and when a woman makes love to her male partner, she is making love to all men (to masculinity personified). This is consistent with tantric beliefs (Anand, 1989) and makes it possible to give up the Freedom Illusion. It certainly lessens the attraction of an affair and also makes it less likely that difficulties such as boredom, dissatisfaction and disillusion that arise in the course of a relationship will be attributed to being with 'the wrong woman/man'.

Reading the above, especially the Poppeliers quote, one might conclude that SGT is only applicable to heterosexual couples. Poppeliers would challenge this conclusion, although he does acknowledge that the theoretical explanation is more complicated. The application, curiously, isn't. He distinguishes between physical form and psychological make-up/energy and, to make sense of the application of SGT to same-sex relationships at this life stage, we need to expand what I was saying earlier.

In a heterosexual relationship the partners are each occupying different physical forms, especially at a genital level. This means that the process of comprehending our partner's physical form, together with their experience of it and also its energetic analogue inside ourselves, is the first stage of mutual understanding and acceptance. This can be difficult because it involves loosening our grip on the part of our sexual identity based on our physical form with which we are strongly connected. For a man, the second stage is to be curious about his female partner's energetic masculinity, and for a woman it is to be curious about her male partner's energetic femininity.

In a same-sex couple, the process of understanding and acceptance is similar, but because each partner's physical form is the same, especially at a genital level, the process of understanding and accepting the aspect of one's partner based on that form is comparatively simple. The difficulty could arise when both partners are trying to understand and accept the aspect of their sexual identity, which is different from their physical form, both in themselves and each other.

In the SGT model, the curiosity and excitement at this stage is focused on exploring the masculine and feminine polarity both internally and in the relationship, the result being a state of wholeness. This exploration can be facilitated by the relationship with parents and parents-in-law, who, ideally, have explored their own and each other's masculinity and femininity and are able to reflect this in their relationship with their grown-up children. The couple can then innocently explore their sexuality together and work towards the experience of wholeness.

Regulation, at this stage, comes both from within the relationship and within the partners themselves. For a man, being grounded in his own masculinity, in balance with his own femininity and recognising his partner as a representative of that femininity means that he is likely to be regulated in his behaviour towards that partner, recognising her as part of himself. Similarly, for a woman, being in balance with her own masculinity, grounded in her own femininity and recognising her partner as a representative of that masculinity means she is less likely to project negative aspects of masculinity onto her partner.

For same-sex couples, the regulation is similar but slightly different. Both partners can identify with each other's masculinity or femininity expressed in their physical form as well as balancing this with their masculinity or femininity expressed and experienced at an energetic level.

Notes

1 Aristophanes proposed the idea that at one time human beings were physically attached in pairs, some both male, some both female and some with one of each. Zeus, fearing that the combined humans were too powerful, decided to separate them, since which time the separated humans have always been looking for their original conjoined partners.

2 In the original, Poppeliers has 'her husband'. I've changed this as much for consistency as anything else.

References

Anand, M. (1989). *The art of sexual ecstasy*. New York: Penguin Putnam Inc.

ONS (Office for National Statistics). (2018). *Birth characteristics in England and Wales: 2018*. Newport: Office for National Statistics. Available at: https://www.ons.gov.uk/peoplepopulationandcommunity/birthsdeathsandmarriages/livebirths/bulletins/birthcharacteristicsinenglandandwales/2018

Perel, E. (2017). *The state of affairs*. London: Yellow Kite.

Plato. (1999). *The symposium*. London: Penguin.

Somé, S. (1997). *The spirit of intimacy*. New York: William Morrow.

Chapter 9

Ripening

This stage begins at 44, a decisive decade for most people in the West and one where it is not uncommon to talk in terms of a 'mid-life crisis'. As the name suggests, the focus in this decade is on the maturing relationship itself, and the work involved in this is that of taking the balancing of masculine and feminine further. Willem Poppeliers talks about 'male femininity' and 'female masculinity' by which he means femininity lived and expressed by someone with a male physical form and masculinity lived and expressed by someone with a female physical form (Poppeliers & Broesterhuizen, 2007).

Clearly, it must be acknowledged that not everyone chooses to be in a relationship at all, much less a committed relationship involving children. Does this mean that Sexual Grounding Therapy (SGT) has nothing to offer them? Thinking about this, bearing in mind the number of participants in SGT that I have encountered who weren't in a relationship when they were involved in the work, I would say that they all had at least a curiosity about why they weren't in a relationship, particularly about why they found it difficult to make and maintain fulfilling relationships. Exploring this question, whether or not this resulted in a change in relationship status, has certainly been important to these kinds of participants.

Willem Poppeliers, curiously, brings the subject of grandchildren into the section of his book which deals with this stage (Poppeliers & Broesterhuizen, 2007). Although this is technically possible, it's much more likely that this might happen towards the end of this decade than at the beginning. It is certain, however, that the children born in the period between their parents' late 20s and mid-30s will be becoming less dependent as the period of this stage (44–54) unfolds and that new children are less likely to arrive during this period.

The other possibility that's becoming very common at this stage is that people may well have separated from their original partner and formed a new relationship, perhaps blending the children of the new relationship with their children from a previous relationship. It may appear, from the discussion of the 'Freedom Illusion' in the previous section, that the SGT stance on this fluidity in relationships is quite old-fashioned. This is probably because an overriding SGT principle at any stage of psychosexual development is to 'put the children at the centre'. This means not only making them a priority in all decisions, including the decision to separate but also recognising that they are at the centre (more correct geometrically 'the apex') of a triangular relationship (see Figure 9.1).

Whilst Willem Poppeliers refutes the negative aspects of Freud's Oedipal triangle, he retains the idea that we are all born into a triangular relationship.[1] We all, even if we are conceived by assisted means, have a biological mother and a biological father, which means that we're born into a triangular relationship, even if that triangle is broken before we come into this world, i.e., one or other parent having left the relationship or died. Somewhere in the universe, that triangle exists with the child at the centre. In thinking about this, we have to be careful making assumptions and judgements, real or implicit, about parents. One good way to do this is to put the child at the centre, focusing on what he/she, as the most vulnerable being in this triangle, needs and wants rather than what the parents should or should not have done.

Children don't judge until they're taught to do so by adults (arguably necessary learning to survive in the real world), but they do know what they need, which in this case is two parents who love each other or can at least relate well enough to enable them to feel safe. As an adult writing this book, I clearly recognise that this isn't always possible and doesn't always happen for a myriad of reasons and it is no part of my intention to judge or criticise the human beings who find themselves in a multiplicity of different, sometimes challenging, roles in relation to the children for whom they are responsible. However, if I put myself into the position of a child, all I know is that I need to feel an important part of a safe triangle and, since it's also important to me to

Mother   Father

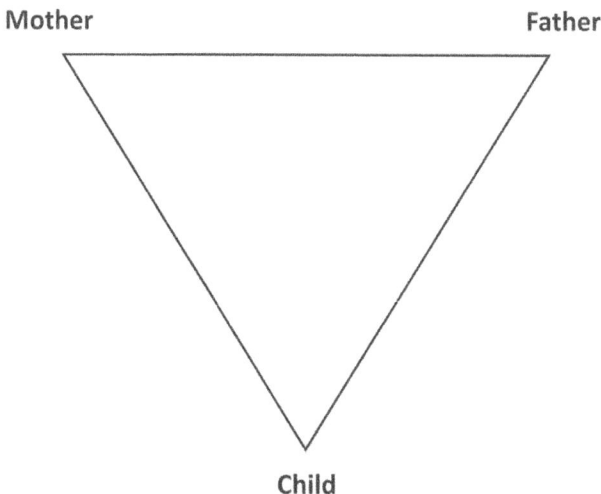

Child

Figure 9.1 The birth triangle

know who I am and where I come from, my biological triangle is crucial to me even if it only turns out to exist in my imagination.

It is important to be precise here. We all have a biological triangle, even if our father was an anonymous sperm donor or a one-night stand. The same holds true if our mother had to give us up for adoption a few days after we were born. However we find out about our origins, we will naturally be curious about them and about our biological heritage and we will almost certainly imagine our missing parent(s). However, it may well get complicated, especially if we are adopted or have step parents. We will then have an emotional triangle as well as a biological triangle and this needs careful handling by the adults involved, which sometimes isn't possible, as notable examples such as *Oranges are Not the Only Fruit* (Winterson, 2014) dramatically illustrate. Aside from the themes of religion and sexuality, which are in themselves interesting from an SGT perspective, the narrator's biological parents hardly feature in the narrative and her purpose in life seems to be to fulfil her mother's wish to have a child without sin. The SGT approach would be much closer to contemporary practice, i.e., putting the child's need to be aware of, and in some cases maintain contact with, their birth parents at the centre of the process.

SGT is, as is becoming clear in this account of the model, a controversial therapy and, when it raises uncomfortable ideas like this, it is tempting to respond defensively. However, Willem Poppeliers is concerned with what he sees as human beings' psychosexual developmental needs and the consequences of their not being met optimally. This is entirely appropriate for a therapist whose model espouses the idea of the reparative therapeutic relationship. Otherwise, the reparation that forms the therapy, and that I shall discuss in more detail later in Chapter 12, may lack the specificity and focus to be effective. The *reasons* for the sub-optimal meeting of developmental needs are less important than the consequences. In the work itself, it is important to acknowledge the incompleteness of the biological triangles in participants' lives and to include triangles consisting of adoptive parents, step-parents etc., according to the need of the participant, in the therapeutic work (see Figure 9.2).

To return to the life stage itself, Willem Poppeliers sees the role of parents and parents-in-law partly in terms of modelling the masculinity/femininity balance and partly as a means of regulating the upbringing of the grandchildren. With our children becoming more independent, and therefore more challenging, issues about how we ourselves were treated when we were our children's age will perhaps be triggered. If parents are able to be open and authentic about the way they treated their children, who are now parents themselves, when they were young, they can support them in being the best parents they can be. Acknowledging their mistakes can be very healing and can also enable their children, as parents themselves, to feel less pressured. They then don't get into the trap of trying to be better parents than *their* parents were and, in the process, becoming more interested in this at an unconscious ego level than in the

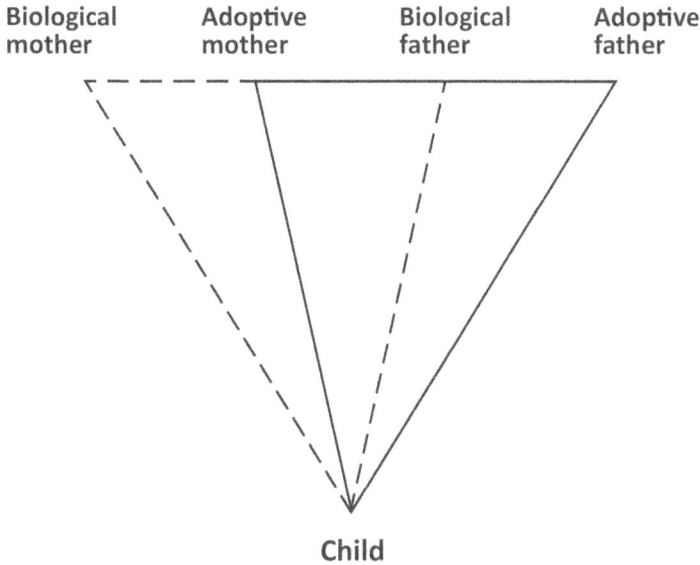

Figure 9.2 The adoptive triangle

welfare of their own children. Often, we can end up projecting our own needs as children onto our actual children. One way of avoiding this is to look after our own inner children, which is one of the aims of SGT work at the earlier stages of development. Internalising our ideal parents enables us to feel that our inner children are now taken care of so that we are then less likely to project them onto our actual children.

Where separated and blended families are concerned, ideal grandparents could well provide a holding role, having less personal interest in the conflict than their offspring and ensuring that the children are central in all considerations.

Note

1 He believes that this holds true even on a cellular level, i.e., that in each cell of our body the triangle we are born into is represented by the DNA from each of our biological parents (W. Poppeliers, personal communication, 2020).

References

Poppeliers, W., & Broesterhuizen, M. (2007). *Sexual grounding therapy*. Breda: Protocol Media Productions.

Winterson, J. (2014). *Oranges are not the only fruit*. London: Vintage.

Chapter 10

Ageing

During this decade, from 54 to 64, two significant things are likely to happen. Our children will, hopefully, become independent and our parents more dependent: one of them may well die during this period. Our parents' ageing and impending death means that they become less and less available to us as sexual sources ideally modelling how to live as sexual beings and, at the very least, as 'anchors'. Even if our contact with them is minimal, we still know that they exist in the physical world, and this provides a stability to our emotional world.

Children will be very likely to have left home during this period and, especially if they have become the focus for much of our emotional energy and attention, will leave a gap, the 'empty nest', when they do so. If they have become too much of a psychosexual focus, as I have described in the chapter on Puberty and Adolescence, this can be very destabilising for their parents' relationship. At the very least, the grown-up children leaving pushes parents in the direction of considering their relationship and the reasons for staying together other than to bring up the children. It can expose the issues between the couple that have been masked by that common purpose, which they then either have to sort out or find another way to obscure. Many of the couples I see in my practice, not necessarily at this stage of life, are effectively saying something like 'We're great parents, but our relationship is rubbish' in their intake questionnaires. Of course, Willem Poppeliers would say that these two things are not separate and that having a vibrant sexual relationship is a vital part of being a good parent.

Relationships can certainly come under a strain during this period, partly because of the 'empty nest' but also because of physiological and psychological changes. Most women will have gone through menopause by this time and both men and women will, however much they wish to deny it, have begun to age, and their bodies will be slowing down. These processes are analogous with psychological equivalents which affect our self-image and psychosexual changes, all of which have an effect of our relationships. Denial is a seductive option, but the challenge, at this stage, is to surrender to the slowing down process, especially as far as making love is concerned (see Richardson, 2011), and to spend time paying attention to our relationship, taking advantage of the time and space in our lives that was previously occupied by our offspring.

Ideally, of course, we will have had the example of our own parents continuing their lives together as sexual beings when we ourselves became independent, and this would mean that we would have been taking care of our relationship in the way described in the last two chapters, but this is rare.

The impending death of at least one of our parents during this decade is challenging, especially on a psychosexual level and if our parents haven't been able to mirror us optimally in the previous developmental stages. In writing this, and having reached this stage of psychosexual development in my narrative, it feels as if I'm getting further and further from many people's lived experience. As the stages pile on top of each other, it can seem that there are so many points at which things can go wrong (I prefer to say that they are 'sub-optimal') that the SGT vision could be viewed as quite pessimistic. A better way to understand this would be to go back to the idea of a therapeutic developmental model's purpose being to highlight what parts of an ideal development are commonly missed in order to be able to re-create them in the reparative situation.

Returning to the decade under discussion, with one parent likely to be dead, there is then a gap in the supportive triangular relationship. This balance can be restored, according to Poppeliers, by the internalised sexual energy and expression of the deceased parent, both by the grown-up child and their surviving parent. Naturally, this assumes a close relationship between all three participants in the triangle, but we are talking ideal situations here.

As we begin to recognise the significance of death, focusing as SGT uniquely does on its sexual implications, it is hard to avoid venturing into the realms of the transpersonal. Although Poppeliers is clear that he doesn't intend his model to be spiritual, but rather rooted or grounded in the body, he does describe the psychosexual stages as being grouped into three different types of paradise (see Figure 10.1).

- 'Paradise in reality' refers to the fact that, given appropriate support and mirroring, the experience of the revealing and development of ourselves as sexual beings is joyous and wonderful.
- 'Paradise in relationship' highlights the potential of sexual relationships to be equally blissful.
- 'Paradise in the generations' refers to the joy of passing support, wisdom, etc. to the generations that come after us in order to support them as sexual beings.

Poppeliers is clear, though, that the paradise he's referring to has a small 'p' rather than large (mine are grammatical!). In other words, he's trying to convey the fact that being connected with your sexuality and living it freely can be joyful, perhaps blissful even, but it certainly needn't involve spiritual beliefs.

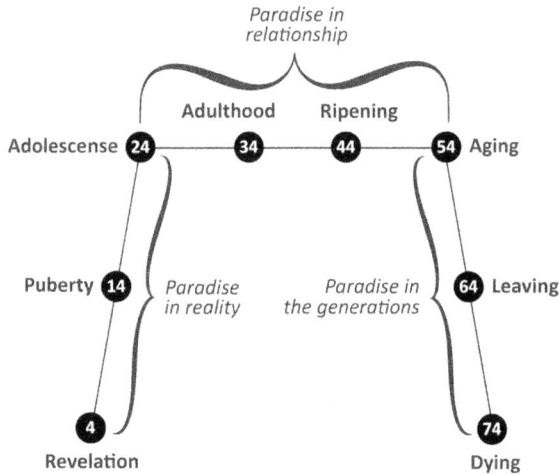

Figure 10.1 Three kinds of paradise

This is similar to the concept of 'Heaven on Earth' expressed by Don Miguel Ruiz (2008) in *The Four Agreements*.

In the same way, in this decade of psychosexual development, Poppeliers also talks about the sexual energy of the deceased parent being free and available and about that parent being available but not in a physical form. Again, whilst he is aware that this way of talking *could* have religious implications, he is clear that it is how we *think* of our parents and their sexual energy that is the important thing, rather than their survival after death in whatever form.

One of the functions of parents at this age, according to Poppeliers, is to teach us how to die and how to let go of our relationships and our sexuality within the context of our past, present and future perspectives. We ourselves can have the opportunity during this decade to clear ourselves of any important unexpressed feelings and parts of ourselves, especially our sexual selves, along with criticisms and resentments we may have been holding onto about our psychosexual upbringing. Clearly this isn't always possible, depending on the circumstances of our parent's death and our relationship with them during this decade, but it can be incredibly cleansing and can also make letting go of that parent a lot easier.

References

Richardson, D. (2011). *Slow sex*. London: O-Books.
Ruiz, M. (2008). *The four agreements*. San Rafael, CA: Amber-Allen Publishing.

Chapter 11

Leaving and dying

During the decade from 64 to 74, with the probable death of our remaining parent, it is impossible not to be aware of our own mortality. The pattern of our parents' deaths has many variations, but often there is a gap between them, which means that we have some time to live with a changed relationship with the surviving parent. This can make it all the more urgent to resolve any relationship issues with them and it can also provide an opportunity for them to offload or share information and stories about their life, which have previously remained hidden. My own father, for example, not only shared information about the woman he'd been involved with prior to marrying my mother but was also quite candid in expressing his regrets about how his relationship with my mother had been. This enabled me to see him much more as the complete, vulnerable sexual being that he was, rather than having a limited perception of who he was and how he experienced his life. I believe the process for him was about reflecting on his life and making sense of it.

All of this makes the internalisation process of the surviving parent's masculine and feminine energy much easier and the experience of that parent's demise, although it is never easy, much less traumatic. If our parents have been 'good enough' we can, at this stage, begin to recognise both the positive and negative aspects of our upbringing, and it is important to do both in order to free up our own energy via our appreciation of our deceased parents as flawed sexual beings. One of the benefits of working through the SGT programme is that we can do this whether or not our parents have been 'good enough', because we will have experienced that 'good enoughness' therapeutically if not in real life.

From our new position in the generation line – the oldest generation in the family along with our siblings – we are reminded of our own mortality and of the importance of our own sexual integrity. In other words, we become aware that we have a limited time in this life and the importance of taking opportunities, especially in our relationship with our partner, becomes paramount.

Although Sexual Grounding Therapy (SGT) regards the Dying stage as the last phase of life, Willem Poppeliers recognises that there is considerable variation in how long it lasts – potentially for more than 20 years. In *Sexual Grounding Therapy* Poppeliers talks extensively about the position of the surviving partner in a relationship (Poppeliers & Broesterhuizen, 2007). In doing this, he is acknowledging the fact that the partner who has died has had to go through a process of letting go of their own life as a sexual being and also of their relationship with the surviving partner. The partner who is left not only has to prepare for their own death but also embody, for their grown-up children, the integration of their two sexual sources and their last link with the older generation.

The idea of 'dying sexually', to use Willem Poppeliers' own words, can sound strange to our ears, but if we accept his original premise that human beings are sexual beings for the whole of their lives, it will perhaps begin to make more sense. We may not necessarily be active sexually for all of our lives, especially in this last phase, but we can appreciate, from a balanced masculine and feminine perspective, the beauty of our own ripened body as well as the bodies of all ages around us. We occupy the position of true elders in our families and communities, even though this may not be appreciated in our culture and, due to our balance and our lack of agenda (we're not trying to prove anything anymore), we are in a perfect place to offer support and advice to children and grandchildren.

Even though our own parents are no longer physically present, they are with us as internalised 'objects'. They have taught us many things in life, either explicitly or by example, the last of which is how to die. When I say this, I'm not so much talking about the act of dying itself, although this might exemplify what needs to be taught, but how to let go and surrender. Of course, what often gets in the way of this is the fear and control that are underlying themes of this book. We can, as I've said, give support and advice to the next generation, but we can't control what they will do with it. We have to trust them to take care of themselves and of the world.

Eventually, we all have to let go of life and Willem Poppeliers' view is that this becomes easier from a balanced position that acknowledges our own loss or as he puts it, 'Dying to the masculinity in the world and dying to the femininity in the world and to the relationship between them' (W. Poppeliers, personal communication, 2020). At peace and in harmony with ourselves, we can embrace our next transition.

Conclusion to the stages

If we look at Willem Poppeliers' eight-stage model of psychosexual development, one thing that stands out is that parents are important not just when we are children but throughout our lives, from birth to death. More specifically, the (Oedipal) triangle into which we're all born is never 'resolved'. It doesn't have to be since it is, in Poppeliers' version, a positive, stabilising relationship. However, it continues throughout our lives to operate in a manner that changes according to the developmental stage we've reached. This isn't the same as saying that we remain *dependent* on our parents for the whole of our lives.

One of the essential premises of SGT is that we are working with the internalised versions of our parents that we carry around with us and that sometimes (often) cause us problems. One of the things I tell clients in all of my therapeutic work is that actual parents (in the here and now of our adult lives) are rarely the problem. The goal of SGT, and all of the other therapy with which I'm involved, is not to change participants' actual parents. This is not an uncommon stance in therapy because we can only work with the person in front of us. In SGT, participants' relationships with their parents *do* change for a number of reasons. Becoming aware of our parents as human beings who both enjoy and struggle with intimacy, sex and relationships will inevitably change the way we relate to them in the present day. Many parents will respond to this, but this is almost certainly because we don't *need* them to.

When we internalise (introject?) our parents, the version we internalise is always a combination of idealisations and demonizations. Although it is probably impossible to eliminate all of these introjections, the work of SGT is designed to enable participants to explore and modify these versions of our parents whilst at the same time working towards an understanding of the two vulnerable human beings who brought us into this world. How this operates in practice will be discussed in the next chapter.

References

Poppeliers, W., & Broesterhuizen, M. (2007). *Sexual grounding therapy*. Breda: Protocol Media Productions.

Chapter 12

The application of the model

Sexual Grounding Therapy (SGT) is a bodywork therapy and so, in its application, the emphasis is on the body and bodily energy. In this it is no different from the Reichian and bioenergetic work from which it is derived. However, unlike these two therapy models, dance is used to promote the circulation of energy in the body and to get participants in touch with their bodies on an emotional and energetic level. When I was involved in Bioenergetics in the 1970s, we used to use movement (a lot of running) and stress positions (Lowen & Lowen, 1977) in order to promote the flow of energy and to work through emotional and physical blocks. In its use of dance, SGT is quite similar to Tantra (my experience of it at least) and perhaps also represents a return to indigenous cultures, who use dance in their rituals to get in touch with their bodily energy, and also with our own culture, where dance serves the function of not only stimulating sexual energy but also bringing potential sexual partners together.

However, the use of dance in SGT is not limited to 'warm-ups'; it can also form an integral part of an exercise or structure. Sometimes 'integral' is an important word in that dance can be used as a way of polarising energy, masculine and feminine, and integrating it. The polarisation between heart and genitals and their integration can also be explored using dance. I invite you, the reader, to try this next time you find yourself on the dance floor (or you could do this in the privacy of your own living room!):

> Dance alone or with a partner, focusing your awareness on the area of your heart. Then, in the next number, perhaps, dance with your focus on your genitals. What do you notice about your movements, about how you feel? What does your partner (if you are dancing with one) notice?

Another technique that is used a lot in SGT is role-play, specifically the (Oedipal) triangle of mother, father, child. As I said at the end of the last chapter, Willem Poppeliers believes that we are all born into a triangular relationship with our parents, whether or not we even know either of them, and that we live emotionally in this triangular relationship for the whole of our lives, however aware of it we may be. These triangular role plays are therefore a feature of the SGT work during all of the developmental stages. As with Family Constellation work with which SGT shares this emphasis, there is much personal insight to be shared, whether you are at the apex of the triangle or at one of the other points as a parent.

In the coursework, there are specific structures that involve the whole group divided into triangles and working simultaneously on the same issue, for example, that of getting the mirroring response you wanted from your parents when you were an adolescent. The triangular role plays are also particularly important in process work when a participant brings a specific life situation into either one of the coursework groups or a sub-group. A good example of this is Josephine,[1] a participant in a sub-group I was leading a few years ago.

Josephine and I were working on the Adolescent stage of development and one of the principles in SGT is that, in working through the psycho-sexual stages, you encourage the client to explore how the life problem that may be occurring in the client's current life looks from the perspective of the stage you're working with in the coursework. Josephine had an ongoing issue with her mother, with whom she was very angry, in her present-day relationship with her. I encouraged Josephine to feel the anger in her body as a 15 or 16-year-old, and when she was able to do this, to choose two people in the group to be her mother and father. She did this and we asked the two people to come and stand in the middle of the group opposite Josephine. I asked her to breathe into her body as a 15-year-old and to notice how she felt when her 'parents' came into the middle and we worked slowly from there.

Eventually it emerged that Josephine, as an adolescent, was experiencing her mother as overprotective, not wanting to recognise her emerging sexuality or allow her any freedom to explore it. She was angry about this and began to express it. I encouraged Josephine's 'mother' to feel, at a body level, what was going on for her[2] in her relationship with her 'daughter', and because it felt as if she was coming from the position of a frightened adolescent girl herself and projecting that fear onto Josephine, I encouraged her to choose a mother for herself in order to feel safe. I asked Josephine's 'grandmother' to stand behind her 'daughter' (Josephine's 'mother'), making physical contact with her.

I then asked Josephine how she was experiencing this on a body level. She said she felt much more relaxed and able to feel and express her own sexual energy without taking responsibility for her mother's fear/control. With her 'mother' behind her, Josephine's 'mother' was able to mirror this energy back to her 'daughter' in a supportive way because she felt safe and supported as a sexual being by her own 'mother', becoming, as I describe in the chapter exploring the Puberty/Adolescent stage, a woman who could say 'yes' to sex as well as someone who could say 'no'. From that position she was able to teach her 'daughter' how to keep herself safe without criticising or controlling her. We went on to explore Josephine's relationship with her father with regard to her emerging Adolescent sexuality, which involved both parents' relationship with each other. This, without going into a lot of detail, resulted in Josephine feeling held and recognised by both parents as the attractive young woman that she was. In her day-to-day life, Josephine became both more understanding of her mother and able to ask for the consideration and recognition she deserved from both parents as a grown-up woman and, more importantly, to behave as if she deserves these in the world.

The above case vignette illustrates how SGT links past experience and present-day issues. The early developmental stages are pivotal in that they frequently establish a pattern that continues to be lived out in our relational lives. We continue to develop physically into adults, but relationally and sexually, we live as uncertain adolescents or even as 6-year-olds.

I described the work earlier in the chapter as 'reparative', and this needs some unpacking, especially since this term has been used to describe a type of therapy designed to change peoples' sexual orientation (Mountford, 2014) with which no Sexual Grounding therapist or trainer would in any circumstances agree. It is tempting, not only to the reader but also to participants who are role playing parents, to imagine this 'reparation' as providing a perfect experience to participants who are in the son or daughter role by giving them what they need, sometimes even without them having to ask. In the work, I frequently need to remind role-playing parents that their job is just to be there and to let the participant who is in the son/daughter role do the work.

The *internal* change is brought about not by giving the client what he/she needs, although this can sometimes happen, but by supporting their impulse to ask for what they need and being there to acknowledge it. In doing this, we are effectively reprogramming the client's body to follow the impulse to reach out for the contact they need and to feel the pleasure in doing this. This principle bears a resemblance to the idea of 'corrective provision', which Martha Stark (1999) explores in *Modes of Therapeutic Action* and which she sees as being influenced by the Object Relations school of psychodynamic therapy. It is also very similar to some of Lowen's bioenergetic exercises, with which I am very familiar (Lowen & Lowen, 1997).

The important thing in SGT is that the flow is from the person in the child role to the person in the parent role and not the other way around. Thus, in the case vignette, Josephine is asking her mother to grow up and be a mother rather than the frightened adolescent, which she normally masks with her defensive veneer of controlling behaviour. Of course, *she* needs *her* mother in order to do this, and one of the powerful aspects of SGT is the instantaneous nature of this kind of transformation at a body level not only of the experience of the 'daughter' but also of the 'mother'. Note that Josephine physically responds immediately when her 'grandmother' comes into the circle and stands behind her 'mother' and before she is consciously aware of what's changed.

One of the ways in which this work becomes powerful is the fact that this kind of role play can be done with the participants naked (I didn't specify this because, as I said, the vignette was an amalgam of different pieces of work I've done over the years some of which have been done naked and others haven't). The choice, in process work like this, rests with the participant whose work it is, but it becomes powerful and is usually gently encouraged because then it's simply not possible for the sexuality, specifically the genitals, of all of the participants to be ignored.

This has different levels. At the level of the role play itself, whilst most people as adults recognise intellectually that their parents possess genitals and have sex, it's challenging for most of us to think consciously about this. I've often encountered this when I've done presentations about SGT and introductory workshops, where I've asked people to imagine their parents having the sex that produced them. The responses are usually along the lines of 'Ewwww' and 'That's weird'! Freud would perhaps attribute this to either repressed Oedipal longings or else to some kind of incest taboo. In SGT, this is seen as a function of the sex-negative culture in which we live, and participants' experience is that this response is something that changes as the coursework progresses and becomes part of the healing experience.

As the reader, it might be useful and interesting for you to reflect on how the above paragraph 'lands' with you:

> Maybe close your eyes and imagine how it might be to be consciously aware of having two parents who had/have sex. How do you think they might do it? What might they like/not like to do with each other sexually? If they're alive, do they still do it? Really take some time to be aware of these questions and of the answers which come to you. Open your eyes again. How was it to imagine and ask yourself these questions? How do you think it might be to walk around in the world, thinking about yourself as the son/daughter of such a sexy mum and dad?

In a role play such as I have described, standing in front of your 'parents' and recognising that they are sexual beings with longings and desires is necessarily challenging, but its directness also has an impact at a body level that bypasses not only the conscious mind but also, with support and guidance, the unconscious defences. As I mentioned at the end of the last chapter, part of the work of SGT involves letting go of both the idealised and demonised aspects of our parents that we've internalised and that are causing us endless problems in our present day lives and relationships. Seeing them naked in a role play enables us not only to take a distance from our internalised images but also to recognise the two people standing in front of us both as the vulnerable, exciting sexy, dynamic human beings that they are and the embodiment, in the role play, of our parents.

At a personal level, there is something important about not hiding your sexuality and your identity as a sexual being from yourself and being open with it towards your 'parents' and asking for recognition and affirmation from them for this important aspect of your being. This can of course be done at an emotional level, even at an energetic level, with clothes on, but it is so much more natural, direct and powerful without. The unequivocal message is: 'I want you to see me, all of me, and to affirm me as the sexual young man/woman that I am!'

At this point, it needs to be made clear that Willem Poppeliers is not advocating the idea that the parents of adolescents should all become naturists in order that their offspring can develop a healthy sexual self-image, although being comfortable with their own naked bodies and their children's at the Revelation stage would certainly establish a good foundation of sexual health.

In real life, it *is* the emotional and energetic level that is important, especially when children reach their teens and become self-conscious about their own and others' bodies. In the family, after all, this is the stage where teenagers start closing their bedroom doors and locking the bathroom door! In therapy though, (most therapy, I would argue) and particularly in this type of workshop format, we're often trying to undo many years of ongoing negative introjections in a one-off experience that needs to be powerful enough to do the job, and this means that the therapy experience is likely to be 'larger than life'. This happens in different ways in different therapeutic models, but in SGT, one way this happens is by working naked.

Working naked is particularly important during the work on the Oedipal phase as this is the age at which we can start to feel embarrassed about or ashamed of our bodies, especially our genitals, particularly when we receive a negative response from our parents at this age. It is also an age where children naturally want to be naked and show off their genitals, as I describe in Chapter 5, in order to elicit the positive response they need. Reading through some of my process notes from sub-group work I have done, I'm struck by how much genital shame there is, especially amongst women, which has its origins in this stage of life, although teenage exposure to the unrealistic depictions of female genitals in pornography also has a part to play. I have also noticed this in discussions with fellow sexuality professionals. What I've noticed in men is that it's not so much the presence of shame as the absence of pride, which can become transmuted into all sorts of negative competition in later life. Another issue that arises very powerfully in the SGT work at the Revelation stage is the number of women whose fathers were, according to the participants' subjective experience at least, disappointed that they weren't boys. There are also significant numbers of men whose mothers wanted them to be girls, but from what has emerged in my experience of SGT work, the disappointment tends to be less overt.

Many of the 'non-mainstream' ways of working with psychosexual issues I described earlier do recognise and work with these issues, especially genital shame, and some of them work with clients naked in order to do this, but, apart from Pelvic-Heart Integration, they tend to work on an adult to adult level. In SGT, there is always a transferential context to the naked work, participants nearly always being in the role of parents, family members or sons/daughters.

The combination of psychotherapy and nudity, apart from some short-lived experiments in the 1960s and early 1970s, is extremely unusual, perhaps because of the transference and counter-transference involved. As I said in Chapter 3, Willem Poppeliers developed SGT as a group therapy in order to lessen the intensity of these unconscious processes, but there are other safeguards in place. The first is that, since SGT therapists are trained professionals, they should be expected to be able to regulate their feelings in the face of participants' nudity much in the same way as they contain their responses to other forms of (erotic) transference and counter-transference.

They should also, like members of the medical profession, be able to look at participants' bodies professionally, i.e., noticing where there is tension or where energy is moving as with any other kind of body psychotherapy. It is important that SGT therapists and trainers respond to participants in a way that enables them to learn that genitals are just another part of the human body, albeit with a vitally important function in sexual relationships. This runs counter to society's fetishisation of body parts, especially genitals, which become, in object relations terms, 'part objects' rather than being integrated into the physical human being. Above all, it is important to re-emphasise that working naked is used in SGT in the service of clients' healing and self-development and within carefully controlled guidelines, which I will discuss in the next chapter.

One aspect of the application of the SGT model that it might be important to address is the age of the participants and how that affects the work. In my experience, as a participant in training and in practice, the age range of participants is from early 30s to early 70s with the highest concentration in the 40s and 50s.

The age of participants is clearly going to affect the nature of their participation. Everyone is going to be doing some looking back and reparation/corrective provision, but, as the coursework proceeds in Part 2, more and more of the participants are going to be looking forward, projecting themselves into the future and preparing themselves for the ageing process (in SGT we prefer to use the word 'Ripening') and ultimately for their death. This is unlike the majority of psychotherapies where the emphasis is on making sense of the past, healing the wounds and/or learning to make different decisions from the ones we made, consciously or unconsciously, in our history and that no longer work for us.

There may be a few other psychotherapies that work in this way. In September 2018, at the conference of the European Association for Body Psychotherapy in Berlin, I was privileged to meet Jeanne Denney, whose School of Unusual Life Learning (SoULL) programme is designed enable practitioners to help their clients to embrace their own deaths.[3] *She* seemed surprised that there were therapeutic models other than her own that worked progressively (i.e., looking forward) as opposed to regressively (i.e., looking backwards as most therapies do) and that included death as part of life to look forward to rather than bereavement as something that needed to be coped with, so it doesn't sound as if there are many approaches that do this.

The SoULL programme is based on a bodywork approach (Denney's background is in core energetics and Somatic Experiencing); however, one difference between the SoULL programme and SGT is that SGT is concerned with all of the stages of life and focused clearly on the *psychosexual* stages. In other words, the therapy is more or less progressive according to the age of the participant with every stage after the one you're chronologically at being a form of preparation for when you reach that stage.

My own experience of this, having gone into the programme at age 54, is that I certainly handled the death of my father very differently (I was 64 when he died) than I think I would have done had I not had this experience. I was fortunate enough to be with him during his dying process and the whole experience felt like more of a privilege than the trauma that it could have been.

Another concept in SGT, which I've already mentioned, is that of 'ideal' parents. As will be clear from my description of the model, most of us have experienced less than ideal parenting, especially in the area of sex and intimacy, and I have already described how, in the SGT work, ideal parents are used in the role plays to enable participants to express and fulfil the needs they weren't able to express at the appropriate age. This is particularly important at the early developmental stages where their internalisation provides a good foundation, or grounding, for the developmental stages that follow. However, the separation between 'real' parents and 'ideal' parents is never as clear as it might seem.

So, for example, in Josephine's work, which was taking place at the Puberty/ Adolescence stage of development, we started with her real parents, specifically her real mother with whom she was very angry. However, simply by being there to receive Josephine's anger, rather than justifying, disputing or even getting angry herself, her mother has moved a long way towards becoming ideal. As the SGT coursework progresses, as the adult stages become the focus, the real and ideal parents become more merged to the extent that, for example, my ideal father becomes the man that my father would have wanted to be and might well have been if he himself had ideal parents. From this position, at the very least a rapprochement, if not forgiveness, is possible either with actual parents, if they are alive, or their memory if they are not. Either way this process is incredibly healing. Instead of projecting our parents onto our partners and others we relate to and experiencing the anger and disappointment that belongs in our childhood in present day relationships, we can feel the support of our parents behind us, which is vital, especially when our present-day relationships become difficult.

Another tool SGT shares with Tantra and Family Constellation work is working with generation lines. These are used both in structured exercises within the week-long workshops and also in process work. Elders are not as revered in our culture as in tribal cultures and the idea of 'ancestor worship', which European settlers encountered in some of the cultures they colonised, was anathema to them. However, there is a fascination at the present time with researching our family trees and some people even send off a DNA sample to find out more about their ancestors. We are arguably more 'connected' than human beings ever have been, but there is still a hunger to know where we come from, where we belong. In Josephine's work, when her mother's mother was brought into the role play, there was the beginnings of a generation line, a line of women going back into pre-history.

Imagining and physically experiencing a line of ancestors behind you, all of whom have lived through broadly similar issues to those you are encountering in your own life, can be really powerful. Naturally the context in which those issues are experienced will be very different, but all human beings have the experience of developing from children into young men and women, making relationships or choosing not to, having children or not, maturing, ripening and dying. Whilst it's clear that the circumstances of each generation are different, with markedly different external influences, pressures and social systems, at the basic level of our human needs, desires and experiences of intimacy, we are not so very different from our ancestors.

I invite you, the reader, to try an experiment.

> Close your eyes and imagine, if you are a woman, your mother behind you and her mother and her mother and her mother, as far back as you can imagine. If you are a man, do the same, but with your father, his father and his father, etc. If you're sitting (I'm assuming most people are when they read), lean back in your chair and imagine that, instead of the chair, your parent of the same sex is supporting you and their parent is supporting them and so on. Breathe and become aware of what this feels like in your body, being physically supported by a whole line of your ancestors.

It would be wonderful to be able to ask you, right now, what you experienced, and I'm also aware that, for some people this may have felt like a strange thing to do. I have to leave that with you to make your own sense of the exercise. However, in the context of SGT workshops, I have observed the effect of being in a generation line as very powerful, and it is used at different stages of the coursework and in the process work as a potent healing tool.

In this chapter, I've given a brief account of the way that the SGT model is put into practice and some of the techniques involved. It gives a flavour of the work and an insight into what a participant might experience during the coursework. Some of the ideas and techniques may be familiar and some may be applicable in other therapeutic contexts. The full experience of SGT is, as I've indicated, very powerful and needs to take place in a safe container, which I shall describe in the following chapter.

Notes

1 'Josephine' is an amalgamation of several different pieces of sub-group work.
2 This is a similarity with Family Constellation work where people who are playing a role are asked what feelings come up for them in that role. It is always surprising (or maybe not) how relevant role players felt responses are to the process that is being explored. In SGT we would, and I did, check out with the person 'working' whether their parent may have responded in the way the role player was responding. I usually find a good correlation here.
3 See www.jeannedenney.com.

References

Lowen, A., & Lowen, L. (1977). *The way to vibrant health*. New York: Harper & Row.
Mountford, C. (2014). 'What a tangled web we weave: Contextualising debate about "reparative therapy"'. *Self & Society*, 42(1–2), 44–51.
Stark, M. (1999). *Modes of therapeutic action*. New York: Aronson.

The organisation and delivery of SGT coursework – the safe container

The coursework is delivered over a period of 2 to 3 years, which clearly represents a substantial commitment for both staff and participants. Although the work focuses on the whole of our lives, the early years, unsurprisingly, receive much more attention and time than the period of adulthood. However, the inclusion of participants' lives as adults is, as I've indicated in previous chapters, a unique feature of Sexual Grounding Therapy (SGT). It is only relatively recently, and in the West, that parents and extended families have been thought unimportant to the psychological well-being of human beings in their adult years. In bringing the positive aspects of life-long parental involvement, especially to our sexual development and maturation, into the therapeutic arena, Willem Poppeliers is arguably taking us back to an era or culture that I described at the beginning of the first chapter.

To return to the structure of SGT, the coursework consists of eight, week-long, residential workshops or blocks, each of which focuses on a psychosexual developmental stage as detailed in this part of the book. These eight blocks are divided into two series, the first four, Coursework 1, being focussed on the period between the ages 4 and 24. It should be re-emphasised at this point that the ages given here are necessarily approximate rather than prescriptive. The second four blocks, Coursework 2, cover the ages between 24 and, in Poppeliers' original design, 74, although, with increased longevity this last is now regarded as somewhat more elastic. Between each block there are small process groups, known as sub-groups, which are an opportunity for individuals to process the learning from each block.

Although there is opportunity for some individuals to process issues that arise for them during the coursework's exercises and structures, it is important that everyone has the chance to process and absorb their learning at a physical and emotional level with appropriate individual attention. Each person can, in the sub-group, work on whatever came up for them either in the previous block or in taking their learning into their personal life afterwards.

This eight-block structure with eight sub-groups represents a container for the exploration of the dynamics/issues that emerge in the course of the work. As I discuss elsewhere in this book, one of the important factors in working explicitly with sexuality is that participants feel safe, and a clear, firm structure is important.

The idea of clients feeling safe is very common across the therapeutic profession these days, but there are different ways both of understanding what this means and of achieving it. In our present-day Western culture, safety is often associated with the complete avoidance of risk. This may sound like 'common sense', but it is both impossible to achieve in reality and not good for us as developing human beings. What is important for children and, by implication, for clients,[1] is to create an overall safe physical and emotional structure in which they can live, whilst at the same time allowing them and encouraging them to explore their physical and emotional impulses within that safe container. In the therapy environment, this is best epitomised by Fritz Perls' description, during the famous 'Gloria' video,[2] of a therapy session as a 'safe emergency'!

In SGT, this safe container is constructed in a number of different ways. First, in most of the countries in which SGT is offered, participants are expected to commit to four blocks at a time (in Mexico, participants are required to commit to both Coursework 1 and Coursework 2 from the start). Apart from the fact that the learning in SGT is cumulative with each block, like the psychosexual developmental stages themselves building on the previous one, it is also important to preserve a sense of consistency for the participants.

Admission to the coursework is subject to attendance at an introductory weekend workshop, which is partly designed to give potential participants a chance to experience the work before making the challenging commitment to embark on the SGT journey. It also gives the SGT staff a chance to see potential participants interacting in a group context so that they are in a position to give informed advice as to whether the programme is suitable for them or not (see my description of SGT as a 'post-graduate therapy' in Part 4). There is, in addition, a comprehensive application form that assists in this process.

This assessment process is important because, as can be seen from my description of the blocks above, SGT starts at the developmental age of 4 to 6, the Oedipal period. This decision reflects Poppeliers' view that, at this age, children begin to discover their own and others' sexuality, begin to notice sameness and difference and begin to relate from the perspective of these discoveries. Clearly, there is an awful lot of psychological development going on before that period and SGT doesn't ignore the enormous significance of this, but it wouldn't see this development as *psychosexual*. Where there are significant issues from the pre-Oedipal period that haven't been explored in other therapeutic contexts, potential participants may be encouraged to do this before committing themselves to the SGT work.

Another component in the creation of the safe container for SGT work is the set of guidelines that all participants sign before commencing the coursework. Apart from what would normally be expected in a therapy contract such as confidentiality, resolutions of complaints, etc., there is clear guidance on sexual boundaries during the work[3] and, in particular and because many participants are also practitioners in their own right, limitations on how participants who have completed the coursework programme can describe their experience on their websites, etc. Our concern here would be about practitioners describing their experience in a way that could be construed by potential clients as indicating that they are trained Sexual Grounding therapists (see the description of the requirements for the latter below).

This leads me on to the final component in the creation of the SGT safe container, the training of Sexual Grounding therapists and trainers. In order to be admitted to the training, prospective trainees need to:

1   Be licensed to practise as psychotherapists (preferably in a body-orientated modality and with some training in unconscious process) in their own country.
2   Have completed Coursework 1 and 2.
3   Complete a comprehensive application form.

To become qualified as SGT therapists they need to complete the training programme – 18 months to 2 years. They are then qualified to facilitate the sub-groups referred to above.

To facilitate the coursework of SGT, therapists have to undertake further training. First, they need to 'shadow' a complete series of coursework modules, observing, taking notes and discussing the material with the trainer. It is expected that they will facilitate sub-groups between the blocks of this coursework. They then have to do the same thing again, this time taking charge of some structures and process work under the supervision of a qualified senior trainer. Once they have done this and fulfilled the various academic requirements of the training, they are then able to facilitate the coursework on their own and are known as 'trainers'.

This nomenclature is slightly confusing to outsiders since participation in the coursework is therapy or personal development rather than training in the conventional sense. The use of the word 'trainer' possibly owes its origins to the fact that, originally, as I said in Chapter 2, the earliest forms of SGT work were a kind of Continuing Professional Development. The expression continues to be used at the moment to distinguish between the competence required to facilitate the two levels of the work – coursework and sub-groups. It may be something that needs to be modified in the future in order to make more sense to the non-SGT community.

Notes

1   As a therapy which has a strong psychodynamic component, SGT makes an equivalence between children and clients who, for therapeutic purposes, are in a regressed state.

2   This is a video that was part of a series of psychotherapy demonstration videos, where one client, Gloria, has a short session with Carl Rogers, Fritz Perls and Albert Ellis. These are now available on YouTube.

3   Not only is sex between participants and trainers strictly forbidden (one would naturally expect this), but sex between participants is also not permitted. Even where participants arrive in a couple, they are strongly advised not to make love during the period of the workshop. This might sound draconian, but given the nature of the mutual transference and regression that occurs during this work, it is believed that participants are not really in a position to make a clear choice and that consent uncluttered by projection and other unconscious processes is not possible.

Conclusion to Part 3

In this part of the book, I've given an account of Willem Poppeliers' Sexual Grounding Therapy (SGT) model. I've explored the psychosexual stages in some detail and explained some of the techniques that are used in its application. I've also described the structure within which Sexual Grounding Therapy is delivered, including the guidelines and the training of SGT therapists and trainers, all of which enable the work to be delivered ethically and safely.

Part 4

Future perspective

Chapter 14

The present and future of the organisation

Currently, the organisation of Sexual Grounding Therapy (SGT) could be described as a franchise. The work is organised by licence holders who pay a percentage of the income generated from running the SGT courses, in the country for which they hold a licence, to the central organisation. This was formerly the Foundation for Sexual Grounding Therapy (FSGT), but we are experimenting with a holacratic way of organising ourselves[1] so this is now known as the Big Circle. The FSGT still exists as the legal entity, having the responsibility, amongst other things, as the awarding body for qualifications in SGT, for liaising with an independent complaints committee and for making links with the scientific world. Some of the revenue generated from the licence holders goes to the founder, Willem Poppeliers, and the rest goes to finance the organisation. Compared with the way in which other models of psychotherapy are organised, this is unusual, but not unique.[2]

As far as the delivery of the work is concerned, the structures and exercises that make up the coursework in SGT were all designed and tested by Willem Poppeliers and, although different trainers, because of time constraints and personal inclination, may decide to include some structures and exercises and leave others out, it isn't expected that they should develop new exercises of their own and include these in coursework calling itself SGT.

Unlike most other models of psychotherapy, SGT is only ever delivered in a group format. Originally, when Poppeliers was developing his ideas, I think he did consider the possibility of using the model in individual sessions, but the intensity of the erotic transference and counter-transference, as has been made clear in Chapter 12, would have made this difficult. Although there may be, inevitably, some transference between the trainer or therapist and the group they're working with, most of the transference is explicitly taking place between the participants, in the process of enacting the roles of parents, grandparents, etc. In this respect, SGT has some similarities with family constellation work, which I've outlined in Chapter 12.

I've also talked, in Chapter 13, about the way that the coursework is delivered, usually over a period of between two and three years as residential workshops with sub-groups in between. Currently, there is a team of Sexual

Grounding trainers and Sexual Grounding therapists delivering Coursework 1 and 2, as well as introductory weekend workshops and sub-groups in France, Germany, Russia, Holland, Mexico, Spain and the UK. Of these, France, Russia and Mexico have ongoing programmes at the time of writing, and the work is in varying stages of evolution in the other countries mentioned. Web addresses for SGT work in all of these countries is contained in the Appendix at the end of the book.

Since all Sexual Grounding therapists and trainers have to be accredited as therapists in their own right before they are admitted to the training and as they are also unique human beings, it is inevitable that each of them will bring their different 'flavour' to the way the work is delivered. The blocks that constitute Coursework 1 and 2 include personal process and theory input, as well as the structures and exercises already mentioned, and this is where the personality and previous experience of each trainer is likely to show itself. However, the overarching developmental schema developed by Willem Poppeliers and described in detail in the introduction to Part 3, together with his exercises and structures, provide a permanent framework within which each individual therapist or trainer carries out the work of SGT.

Organisationally, SGT is in transition and has been for a number of years now. The founder, Willem Poppeliers, has more or less withdrawn from clinical work and is also less involved with the organisation, even though he is still available for consultation as required and takes an active interest in current developments. His focus, as I shall describe later, is now mostly on the scientific side of the work.

When Poppeliers originally developed SGT, he delivered all of the coursework himself under the auspices of Bodymind, as I mentioned in Chapter 2. As the work became more widely known, it not only became obvious that Poppeliers wouldn't be able to deliver all of the coursework himself, but he had also attracted other practitioners who were interested in being trained in this powerful, new and exciting model of psychosexual therapy. My impression is that this first generation of trainees learned 'at the feet of the master', mostly by the apprenticeship model I referred to in Chapter 13.

Looking at it from a historical perspective, this has not been uncommon in the history of psychotherapy although it is unusual now. In Freud's day, you were invited to join his seminar/discussion group and, having presented a paper and contributed to the discussions of others' casework, you would be referred clients by Freud and begin to build your practice (Of course, you needed also to have a medical qualification before being admitted to the seminar group in the first place!).

My own training in psychotherapy was quite similar in that we were certainly learning at the feet of the master, or in this case the mistress, Tricia Scott. She wasn't teaching an entirely original model but her own synthesis of bioenergetic analysis and Reichian bodywork. There's a lot to be said for this style of training. It's definitely live, exciting and directly responsive to the needs of the trainees. You have the feeling that you're at the cutting edge of the work, the curriculum being constantly adapted to both the needs of the trainees and emerging developments. Our assessment was ongoing, direct and responsive not only to our knowledge of theory and technique but also to our ability to internalise and manifest the principles of the work. There are problems though. One difficulty is that this style of training puts a lot of power/responsibility in the hands of the 'master', which can become a burden that is difficult for even the most well-balanced human being to carry. Another problem is that of what happens to the subsequent generations of trainees when the founder takes a back seat, and I think this is what we're dealing with, organisationally, in SGT at the moment.

Many therapeutic organisations don't survive the withdrawal of their founder. The organisation I trained with certainly didn't; although, as I said, the model we were working with wasn't as systematised as the SGT model. This meant that those of us who wanted to continue practising were able to do so under our own auspices when the organisation came to an end, although many chose not to.

Looking into the future, organisationally, the task for SGT is to find a structure that all of us feel able and willing to commit to that enables the work to continue and develop whilst maintaining its combination of freedom and regulation, which is an essential characteristic. One development that has already been achieved is that the training of SGT therapists has been systematised and updated so that its structure resembles a more conventional model of psychotherapy training and also enables trainees to feel regulated and stable. At the same time, it also has enough flexibility to give them the freedom to develop their own individual working style.

The education of SGT trainers still adheres to the apprenticeship model (see Chapter 13), which, from personal experience, I would say is an appropriate model for such advanced learning. The only difficulty is that, because the trainer in education needs to shadow and gain experience in two complete programmes, and those programmes don't necessarily run regularly, it can take a considerable period of time for a trainer to become qualified. Although I'm identifying this as a difficulty, there is a positive side to this situation in that it ensures that those who go on to practice are both well-trained and committed.

In this chapter, I've given a subjective picture of the SGT organisation as it is at the time of writing. As may be obvious, at this stage of the book, I consider the work to be profound, innovative and unique, and I'm confident that it will continue in some form. What that form will be, especially organisationally, is difficult to predict at the present time.

Notes

1 Holacracy is a non-hierarchical, role-based management structure. See www.holacracy.org for more information.

2   There is a rationale for this in SGT. The work is always delivered as a series of pre-scribed structures and exercises, interspersed with process and theoretical input, which are extremely powerful and challenging. The fact that these liberate, at each of the psychosexual stages, the natural excitement, curiosity and innocence that in many of the participants may have been repressed for years, means that it is important that these structures and exercises are delivered in a contained way by practitioners who have been fully trained and are accountable to their peers in the organisation. In this way, the intrinsic desire for regulation from the outside, which is especially appro-priate to the 'opening' phase of psychosexual development, is met. The present franchise structure maintains this regulation, containment and accountability and at the same time recognises the work of the founder, Willem Poppeliers, involved in developing the theory, structures and exercises.

Chapter 15

The clinical future of SGT

Looking into the future, clinically, also has its challenges. My own experience as a participant is perhaps useful here. Before I came to Sexual Grounding Therapy (SGT), I had already undertaken years of one-to-one and group psychotherapy and was trained in Bioenergetic/Reichian therapy and couplework. It seemed to me that SGT was a 'post-graduate' therapy in that it worked at a very deep and challenging level and seemed to reach the parts other therapies I'd experienced hadn't reached, especially in addressing the issues later in life. I'm not sure how I would have responded had I not done any work on myself before coming to my first experience of SGT. Clearly, it's impossible to answer this question definitively, but I have also observed that, in my cohort of participants and in the cohorts I observed during my training, most people had done at least *some* therapy or personal growth activity before coming to SGT.

Given the depth at which SGT works and the fact that it's delivered in 6-day blocks that can be as much as three months apart, it's important that participants have a degree of stability in order to be able to function between the blocks, even when a lot of material may have been stirred up for them. This means that SGT not only demands a considerable commitment from potential participants, but it also may not be suitable as a first therapy, especially for people with significant pre-Oedipal issues (see Chapter 13).

One solution to this issue could be to be explicit that previous therapeutic experience is an essential requirement for admission to the programme. Proposals have been made in the past to address this issue by extending the work to include the pre-Oedipal stages of development. This might have some theoretical support from Kleinian therapists, since Klein is known to have projected the Oedipal stage of development back into early infancy, but, in my opinion, such a move would run the risk of changing the character of the work, from a specifically psychosexual therapy to a more generalised therapeutic model.

Nevertheless, in Russia, the therapeutic team has introduced the idea of a 'pre-Coursework 1' block designed to address some of the pre-Oedipal issues that were otherwise making the coursework difficult there. I think, though, that there is a marked difference between the situation in Russia and that in Western Europe (colleagues have spoken about a collective trauma that pervades the Russian psyche)[1] and, because this method of dealing with the pre-Oedipal issues responds to this difference, it is probably a good solution to the specific problem there.

As my colleague Ingo Vauk has identified in the endnote to this chapter, there is a strong argument for saying that pre-Oedipal issues (i.e., attachment and object relations issues) are best addressed in one-to-one therapy where the client can be allowed to regress and to demand total attention, being mirrored, in the Winnicottian sense of the word, by the therapist, who becomes the client's 'good enough' mother (see Winnicott, 1967; Stark, 1999). This is entirely consistent with Erikson's psychosocial model of development, which assumes that a child's world gradually gets wider as they develop, initially being based solely on the mother-child dyad and expanding outwards to include the whole of humanity.

Whatever solutions we evolve, it remains true that, if participants have unresolved severe disturbance at the pre-Oedipal stage, it can have an effect not only on their own participation in the programme but also on the experience of their fellow participants. My own preference would be to refer such potential participants for intensive one-to-one relational psychotherapy, after which they could be admitted to the SGT programme. In Western Europe, and certainly in the UK with the number of available individual therapists I referred to at the beginning of Part 2, this is comparatively easy. In countries such as Russia, it's not as straightforward, which is another good reason for adopting the strategy that is currently in place there.

Another possible direction for expanding the future work of SGT, which would make the work better known, is 'Applied SGT', i.e., professional development work and/or supervision that uses the fundamental theories of SGT but applies them in the context of one-to-one therapy or couplework. There is some interest, within the organisation, in developing this and there has been good feedback from the workshops we've offered so far in the UK. This feedback has included comments on the paucity of input to mainstream psychotherapy and counselling training courses on psychosexual issues, which I've referred to in Chapter 3. If you are a practitioner reading this book, you may already have come across ideas and concepts that, either consciously or unconsciously, might find their way into your therapeutic practice. Similarly, those of us who have done the SGT coursework programme and the clinical training will inevitably be using some of the concepts and ideas, both in our clinical work and, more importantly, in our supervision.

Another clinical direction, which has already been tried in some places, is the idea of couples' groups, men's groups and women's groups that use SGT principles but are not part of the Coursework 1 and 2 programme. Both this direction and the 'Applied SGT' direction raise the idea of a division between the ideas and concepts of SGT and the Coursework 1 and 2 programme. As far as the former is concerned, we need to be aware, as an organisation, that the full training in SGT represents, as I've said in Chapter 14, a major investment of time, money and energy to which many practitioners, even though they may be interested in the work, may be reluctant to commit. There could thus be an advantage to the SGT organisation in making this separation, which would allow the ideas and concepts, many of which, as may be clear by this point in the book, have their roots and derivations in other therapeutic models, to be freely available to the therapeutic world.

As far as the groupwork based on SGT principles is concerned, it is the making of this separation that is important in itself. In other words, the important thing is to make sure that the exercises and structures which are specific to Coursework 1 and 2 aren't used in any of these groups and that there is no implied equivalence between attendance at these groups and participation in the Coursework programme.

Another important direction in which SGT could take itself would be working with young people between the ages of 18 to 35. In a typical coursework group, we may get one or two people in the upper end of this age range, but most of the participants tend to be middle-aged. Yet the 'millennials' are really struggling, as I've said Chapter 6 and Chapter 7, with identity, relationships, etc. They haven't had the mirroring they need, but they do have a lot more hype and pressure around sex, which is exacerbated by social media and online porn. Véronique/Vasanti is doing some wonderful work in this area in France and last summer's international Impulse Festival,[2] which developed out of the groupwork which Vasanti has been doing over the last 20 years with young people and which makes use of SGT principles amongst its other influences, was a great success. It would be really good to see this developed in other countries.

Notes

1   There are many reasons, in my opinion, why we find working in Russia different to working in the West. There is a lot of collective trauma throughout Russian history, the most obvious and recent in the 20th century: revolution, two big invasive wars, the brutality and injustices of the Stalinist and, generally speaking, the Communist era will have affected almost every family in the states of the former Soviet Union. Since then, there has been the breakup of the system and the painful road to the current political situation, which in itself is not free of traumatic impact.

As SGT therapists, we know about trans-generational issues, so we can see that these collective phenomena have left traces in each and every individual. On the individual level these traumata were to be seen as interrupted family lines, alcoholism running through family systems, violent and sexual abuse and gender roles that are far more archaic than we experience them in the West. Multiple abortions are not uncommon in the generation of our clients' mothers, as well as the women we encounter in the groups.

As SGT touches every individual so existentially, it is obvious that the material will trigger any of these traumata in our clients above and beyond the material contained in the usual SGT work. We therefore thought that it would be good to run a 'Level 0' workshop in order to deal with, and give the clients some tools to handle, such trauma. However, realistically we have come to the conclusion that these issues are too diverse and of a magnitude that cannot be dealt with in a group setting and within the framework of a 6-day workshop.

So, we have decided to run introductory workshops more in order to filter out participants who are not resourced enough to do this deep work just yet and have started to network with trauma therapists who support clients during the course of the SGT program in smaller, more suited groups and individual sessions. This has been implemented in the current program for the first time and, so far, looks very promising (I. Vauk, personal communication, 2020).

2 See www.impulsefestivals.com.

References

Stark, M. (1999). *Modes of therapeutic action*. New York: Aronson.

Winnicott, D. W. (1967). Mirror-role of the mother and family in child development. In P. Lomas (Ed.), *The predicament of the family: A psycho-analytical symposium* (pp. 26–33). London: Hogarth.

Chapter 16

SGT in the world

One of the major issues facing Sexual Grounding Therapy (SGT) in the future is that of where it positions itself in the world. Part of the purpose of this book has been to establish SGT's position, both historically and in relation to other methods of working with sexuality. Where there is a future decision to be made, however, is in whether we want to be part of the mainstream in psychotherapy, or whether we belong on the fringes, part of the non-mainstream I identified in Chapter 4 or, as I think we actually are, somewhere in between these two.

This is not an easy question. On the one hand, it has always been important to Poppeliers that SGT distinguishes itself from unregulated work, such as that of his erstwhile colleague Jack Painter and other contemporary work in the field of sexuality where the boundaries may not be as we would expect them to be in SGT. This pushes us towards the mainstream, and I can certainly see an argument for that position, as I'm sure my colleagues may well do. However, my experience of mainstream psychotherapy in the UK over the last 35 years has not left me with a great inclination to be any more involved with it, organisationally, than is necessary. Again, the issues of control and fear, which have emerged frequently in this book, become important here.

Looking back to the history, Freud's original ideas and the framework within which he looked at sexuality were revolutionary when he was developing them at the end of the 19th century. According to Reich (1973) though, as psychoanalysis became more established as an institution, Freud and those around him diluted a lot of his ideas, and control became more of a factor in his work than exploration and liberation. Reich then became the therapeutic revolutionary and arguably suffered as a consequence. As I've already intimated, it is possibly as a reaction to the dismissal of his radical ideas that he became more and more extreme in his attempts to demonstrate their scientific validity.

Some of the post-Reichians, Lowen for example, definitely became part of the establishment, as I've already observed. Stanley Keleman, in his writing, mostly focused on form, energy and feeling without much reference to the social implications of the therapy he was talking about. The exception to this was his controversial book, *In Defense of Heterosexuality* (Keleman, 1982), where he expresses views that were challenging to the therapeutic ethos of his time and would almost certainly have him 'no platformed' today. More recently, other post-Reichians, notably Nick Totton, have managed to maintain their radical stance. Nick's writing is explicitly political (Totton, 2000) and his work in co-creating the Independent Practitioners Network is a testament to his commitment to remain outside the mainstream, but he is careful to avoid the kind of controversy Keleman created in the book I referred to above.

In looking for an appropriate position in relation to the world, one possibility is to equate the position of the psychotherapist with that of the philosopher in ancient Greece. According to Socrates, the philosopher should occupy the position of a gadfly on the noble steed of the state (Plato, 2002, p. 124).[1] Socrates maintained this position – on the fringes rather than part of the establishment – by refusing to accept financial support from anyone who was not a believer in his precepts. If we, as psychotherapists, are able to maintain the position that Socrates advocates, this will make it much easier to support our clients in challenging the status quo, not only on an internal level, but also socially. This is difficult if the therapy we are delivering is funded and/or regulated by institutions that are part of the social structure that the client may need or wish to challenge.

It is also much more difficult, as a therapist, to challenge both the social and your client's internal status quo if you are constantly worried about how what you're doing fits with not only the medical establishment (which I shall discuss under the heading of SGT and science) but also the prevailing mainstream therapeutic establishment.

My experience of trying to get a Continuing Professional Development (CPD) programme using SGT endorsed by the College of Sexual and Relationship Therapists (COSRT) is an illustration of this. This programme was delivered jointly by the Centre for Gender Psychology and Inter-Psyche (a counselling training organisation of which I was the director and which was run as part of Kent and Medway NHS and Social Care Partnership Trust) and was rejected because I'd mentioned SGT in my description of the course. Someone from the COSRT had discovered that SGT works with clients naked, and I was told that 'the college couldn't possibly endorse anything like that'. I explained that (a) the CPD course wouldn't be working with anyone naked, and (b) we had a detailed set of guidelines that participants in the SGT coursework were required to sign before they were allowed to continue with the work, but to no avail!

To be fair, when any therapy deals as openly with sexual issues as SGT does, there are bound to be assumptions about the work that get treated as fact. One assumption that I've heard is that the therapists (trainers) are naked during the work (they are not) and another is that there is 'hands-on' touch between therapists (trainers) and participants (there is not). Given the way that the press has treated some high-profile cases of therapist sexual misconduct, I can understand the need for caution. However, I can clearly state that, since I became a member of the board of the Foundation for Sexual Grounding Therapy (FSGT), the regulatory board of SGT, in 2007, although we have had a small number of concerns brought to our attention (none of which has become an official complaint) about various aspects of the work, *none* of these has been connected with sexual misconduct. This experience is consistent with Tree Staunton's statement in Chapter 3 of *Body Psychotherapy*: 'There is no evidence to suggest that touch or physical contact with clients [she *is* talking about touch between therapist and client here] increase the likelihood of acting out sexually, nor that distance nor analytic rigour prevent it' (Staunton, 2002, p. 51).

The problem with being accepted into the mainstream is that there is always a price for this, and that usually means being controlled by it. This can, as I explore in my paper 'The Therapist as Gadfly' (Lamb, 2018), effectively eviscerate any therapy that is based on more than restoring clients to a condition of 'normality'. The Improving Access to Psychological Therapies (IAPT) programme in the UK NHS is a prime example of this process. I have the greatest respect for therapists such as Mick Cooper, who worked tirelessly to create a version of person-centred therapy that would fit into the Procrustean bed of the IAPT system.[2] However, I can't see how a 'treatment', which in practice can be for as few as three sessions (Scott, 2018), a significant proportion of which are taken up with psychometric testing, and which Scott regards as contaminating the accuracy of the test in any case, can enable a client to reach the level of self-awareness/self-worth, etc. envisaged by Carl Rogers (2003) when he developed the person-centred model.

One of the concepts in SGT that supports the challenging of the social status quo is that of 'surplus value'. When you have internalised your parents and their affirmation of you as a sexual being, you approach your relationships from the position of having something – your 'surplus value' – to share rather than from a position of need. You are also in a good position to support the next generation. Apart from improving the quality of their relationships, enabling clients to approach their lives from a feeling of 'surplus value' contributes to the subversion of the consumer capitalist system. This system, in order to be successful, requires the population to be in a state of perceived need that they then fulfil by buying consumer products and services. As I remarked in Chapter 1, the establishment also benefits from the population being in a state of fear, which creates a need for, and acceptance of, external control.

When they don't have a grounded (sexual) identity or sense of themselves, people are also more likely to identify with a race or a nation that they can 'make great again', usually by making some other race or nation worse off! When looked at from this perspective, SGT can be seen to be extremely radical, which is a very good reason not to go through whatever process might be required for it to be accepted into the mainstream, unless of course that mainstream itself changes.

Another important issue for SGT in its relationship with the world is that its theory assumes differences between men and women, and this is increasingly questioned in mainstream psychotherapeutic circles as well as some of the non-mainstream circles I explored in Chapter 4. True, we can get around this by talking more about masculinity and femininity, but even this is becoming unacceptable in some contexts.

As a body psychotherapist, I believe that I don't just have a body, but I *am* my body and my body is me, a sentiment that was the topic of a conversation between Sam Keen and Stanley Keleman in the 1970s (Keen, 1973). As I re-read this sentence, I realise that it could be interpreted as mechanistic and I don't mean that. The important idea as far as SGT is concerned is that, although there is a fundamental principle in its theory and practice of balancing masculinity and femininity as a developmental ideal, the fact that I am a male body, that my genitals are male, has a significance. However, in SGT, that significance is limited; it's just about what's immediately, viscerally and energetically available to me. To be sure, I can think about certain body parts that might have a feminine quality (I have quite sensitive hands for example), but to fully experience my femininity, I have to use my (bodily) imagination. The SGT work itself uses guided meditation, movement and dance to facilitate this kind of exploration and balancing.

The problem comes when we attribute unlimited, sometimes irrational significances to our male and female bodies, such as feeling or not feeling certain emotions, being suited to certain jobs, activities or academic disciplines, etc. When power and status become involved, as they inevitably will when you limit certain roles and activities on the basis of genital difference, the situation becomes even more difficult, and battle lines are drawn. We become very preoccupied with whether differences are intrinsic (nature) or whether they're socially conditioned (nurture), the implication in the latter case being that the function of the conditioning is to maintain the power imbalance in favour of the patriarchy. The difficulty is that, whilst there is certainly truth in the latter implication, the preoccupation can itself obstruct our true empowerment as men and women, which starts with being comfortable and grounded in our own bodies.

In SGT, working naked means that it is impossible to ignore sexual differences, as I've already said in Chapter 12, but it also makes it difficult to attribute power or status to those differences – effectively, nobody is 'wearing the trousers'.

Putting the child at the centre as usual, the SGT approach to this difficulty is to look at what all of us as individuals need, as we develop, to feel comfortable with ourselves as sexual beings, whatever our gender. However we may define our sexuality later in life, as children we all need to feel seen, recognised, responded to and accepted as sexual beings, wherever on the spectrum of expressions, behaviours and body shapes, we find ourselves. Once we begin to become socialised, as I've described in Part 3, things get more complicated, and it has to be recognised that the effects of that socialisation are different for each of us as individuals. However, they still come down to the need to be seen, recognised, responded to, and accepted as the unique sexual beings that we are.

This need is something that SGT, in both its theory and practice, uniquely and powerfully supports.

SGT undoubtedly does make reference to men and women, but the significance of those terms is bodily and energetic, as I've described it above. Perhaps, even though it seems slightly cumbersome, we should talk in terms of male bodies and female bodies or even, as seems to be the current practice, vulva owners and penis owners!

If SGT is to practise what it preaches, then we need to approach the world from a position of 'surplus value'. What this means is that we should definitely make the world aware of our existence (this book is a formal step in that direction), but we should always do this from the position of having something to share rather than from a position of need.[3] In this way our relationship with the world is analogous to what we're advocating in a mature evolved sexual relationship.

The SGT organisation, by reason of the requirements of its training programme, is in a unique position in this regard. The condition that trainees are all registered to practise psychotherapy in their own country before embarking on their training means that they are all, in theory at least, able to earn a living in their original model of training and therefore don't need to depend on their earnings as SGT therapists and trainers. It is important that we maintain this stance as an organisation, developing and maintaining our relationship with the world but not changing ourselves to fit in with what we think the world might accept.

Notes

1 'Gadfly' is a generic term for a horsefly and any other insect whose bite can have the effect of disturbing horses or cattle, sometimes causing them to run or stampede.
2 I'm not sure whether Poppeliers was aware, when he used this term, of its Marxist origin, although Marx used the term to indicate the value added to a product by the labour that went into it, most of which was appropriated by capitalists.
3 I would argue that this principle probably applies to all therapists and therapeutic organisations. It may sound strange to talk about therapists approaching the world from a position of need, but in the UK, the emphasis on 'marketing' that I observe in the profession these days certainly looks like need, even if that need is being projected onto potential clients, i.e., persuading them that they need you when the reality is that you need them. I'm grateful to my original trainer, Tricia Scott, for instilling in me the idea that we should never become dependent on our therapy clients, and we should be able to walk away, as she herself did at one point in her career, if it no longer feels right to carry on practising as a therapist.

References

Keen, S. (1973). 'We do not have bodies, we are our bodies'. *Psychology Today*, 7(4), 64–70.
Keleman, S. (1982). *In defense of heterosexuality*. Berkeley: Centre Press.
Lamb, G. (2018). 'The therapist and gadfly'. Available at: http://www.geoff-lamb-psychotherapist.com/article-the-therapist-as-gadfly.html

Plato. (2002). *Five dialogues*. Indianapolis: Hackett.

Reich, W. (1973). *The function of the orgasm*. New York: Noonday Press.

Rogers, C. (2003). *Client centred therapy*. London: Constable.

Scott, M. (2018). 'Improved access to psychological therapies – The need for radical reform'. *Journal of Health Psychology*, 23(9), 1136–1147.

Staunton, T. (2002). *Body psychotherapy*. Hove: Brunner-Routledge.

Totton, N. (2000). *Politics and psychotherapy*. London: Sage.

SGT and science

And so we come to the question of Sexual Grounding Therapy (SGT) and science. My own experience is quite relevant here. Unlike some psychotherapists who study psychology first and then go on to undertake a psychotherapeutic training, I did it the other way around. When my original training organisation came to an end, many of us were looking for future directions and, although I chose to continue to practise as a psychotherapist, I decided to go back to university and study psychology, which mutated into studying neuroscience (it was a modular degree). One of the ideas I was interested in exploring was whether it might be possible to demonstrate scientifically that body psychotherapy had a measurable physiological effect.

I discovered some theoretical support for this possibility in the field of psychoneuroimmunology, which looks at the relationship between psychological processes, the nervous and immune systems. Most studies I came across in this area looked at stress and other causal psychological variables and their effect on the immune system. Theoretically, this represented a possible means of testing the efficacy of psychotherapy by looking at the effect of psychotherapy on these variables as measured by the functioning of the immune system. However, none of the studies I came across seemed to be interested in looking at psychotherapy, except perhaps for Cognitive Behavioural Therapy (CBT). I discussed a possible project with a friendly General Practitioner (GP), who was the husband of a counsellor I had trained. This would have involved doing blood tests on a cohort of patients before and after therapy and looking for biological markers of immune system function. In principle, he was encouraging, but he was doubtful of the feasibility on many practical and ethical grounds.

Another dream I had was to give clients MRI scans before and after significant therapy sessions and look for differences. At the level at which I was studying, access to such facilities was impossible and, in the end, I discovered that the most sentient creature I was allowed to experiment on at undergraduate level was a leech! I also discovered, whilst trying to set up research projects for my master's degree, where I wanted to look at the connection between social emotional support in men and their recovery from myocardial infarction, that recruiting volunteers for this kind of project is fraught with difficulty. Clearly, work like this has a lot of ethical as well as funding implications, and my enthusiasm needed to be channelled in different directions.

More recently, my reading of Terry Lynch's *Beyond Prozac* and Candace Pert's *The Molecules of Emotion* (see Lynch, 2004; Pert, 1999) confirmed for me how dominated medical research is by the pharmaceutical industry and how difficult it is to get support for any experimental work that doesn't fit in with their mainstream ideas. And of course, one of the motivations behind carrying out such research would be to be accepted by the mainstream, which, as I've said in the previous chapter, I feel is of questionable value.

All of this leads to a difficult position with regard to taking SGT work in a more scientific direction. At the moment, the situation could best be described as 'work in progress'. Currently, the Foundation for Sexual Grounding Therapy (FSGT) has a scientific committee consisting of Willem Poppeliers; the President of FSGT, Dr Theo Royers; and Dr R d'Abreu of Radboud University Nijmegen. The committee has put forward two proposals for research projects, one about hypo/hyper-sexual behaviour and the other about the relationship between attachment style and risky (homo)sexual behaviour, neither of which has received sufficient funding to go ahead. In 2016, Willem Poppeliers established a fund in collaboration with the Radboud University whose purpose is to fund future research into SGT. The only disadvantage of this is that the source of funding is a future bequest from Poppeliers himself, which means that the founder of Sexual Grounding won't be able to directly witness the research and its results.

The progress I've identified above is definitely a move in the right direction, and I'm aware that making links between SGT and science is important to Poppeliers at this point in his life. I would also be delighted if a research project could be set up in order to do establish these links. However, my experience and my reading lead me to adopt a more cautious position – I'm not holding my breath. On a more positive note, my own experience both as a mature student and in my more recent reading has been that scientists from other disciplines are definitely receptive to the idea of connecting emotion to physiological process. Scientists on the fringes of the mainstream (Bruce Lipton, Stephen Porges, Iain McGilchrist, Daniel Seigel, etc.) also write in a way that is very sympathetic to the kind of therapeutic work in which we're engaged in SGT. This can feel very encouraging, but it's a long way from getting a project off the ground that would experimentally validate the efficacy of SGT.[1]

We have to remember that these writers are starting from the position of having established a track record in mainstream science and are moving from there to become interested in interventions that might be considered to be on the fringes. In their consideration of these fringe interventions, even the most adventurous scientists such as Pierre Capel (2019), whose latest book investigates the relationship between feelings and DNA, tend to err on the side of caution. Capel starts from the physiological processes he's interested in and in which he has expertise, makes a connection between these and psychological processes and restricts the interventions he discusses to safe areas such as sport, yoga and meditation (Capel, 2019). This is very different from moving in the opposite direction, that is to say taking a controversial therapeutic model and looking for scientific validation of that specific form of intervention.

For the moment, the most useful direction we can go in scientifically is to keep talking to the potentially sympathetic scientists that we meet (Poppeliers is already doing this in Holland), keep a look out for writers like those I have mentioned whose work is in step with ours, and endeavour to build bridges with them without compromising ourselves in the process. One way of achieving the latter would be to not approach this from the position of need I mentioned at the end of the last chapter. It may sound arrogant, but a positive way of expressing this would be to say that the scientists are catching up with what humanity, when it's in touch with itself, has known intuitively for generations.

Note

1 One of the reasons that so little conclusive research into non-CBT models of psychotherapy has been carried out is that most other therapies are difficult to 'operationalise', i.e., to reduce to a standard series of 'inputs' on the part of the therapist. They depend on other uncontrollable variables such as the personality of the therapist delivering the therapy and the quality of the therapeutic relationship as well as on 'client variables' such as the client's commitment to the work, the amount of external support they have in their lives, etc. (see Mearns & Cooper, 2005).

References

Capel, P. (2019). *The emotional DNA*. Amsterdam: K.pl Education.
Lynch, T. (2004). *Beyond Prozac – Healing mental distress*. Ross-on-Wye: PCCS Books.
Mearns, D., & Cooper, M. (2005). *Working at relational depth in psychotherapy and counselling*. London: Sage.
Pert, C. B. (1999). *The molecules of emotion*. New York: Simon & Schuster.

Chapter 18

Ending

I have encountered many challenges in writing this book, and the one I'm facing now is how to end it. As I've been working on it, and through my current work with individuals and couples, I've become more and more aware, not only of the amount of sexual distress there is in our 21st-century world but also the lack of fulfilment that pervades much of our lives, not just in the sexual arena. We are distant, as human beings, from our own bodies, from our intimate partners, from family, friends and most of all from the world we live in. This feeling of separation (Marx might call it 'alienation') is double-edged. On the one hand, it can be attractive, in that it can seem to make our lives a lot less complicated and easier to control. If we're disconnected from those around us, we can sometimes feel less controlled by them – what they think matters less to us so we can do what we like, and then we have the illusion of freedom. We also feel more in control ourselves, because the distance we make lessens our feeling of vulnerability.

On the other hand, separation leads to a diminution of fulfilment. Nothing/no one is important, and there is therefore no pleasure in sharing or closeness, which, on the contrary, can be experienced as a restriction or a threat. Sometimes we believe that the answer to this lack of fulfilment is to seek pleasure through pursuing sensation and excitement rather than through intimacy and relationship. In our sexual relationship, our partner may not wish to join us in our sensation seeking, and this too can be experienced as a restriction, which may in turn cause us to disconnect further. The remarkable thing is that in relationships, although people sometimes, for reasons of their own insecurity, do behave in a controlling manner, this isn't an inevitable result of being close – the opposite in fact. The control is there to make and keep the distance and to preserve the self-perceived fragility of the person doing the controlling.

Another factor that supports the creation and maintenance of this climate of separation is our concern with identity. We have become preoccupied with discovering and expressing ourselves, which isn't a problem in itself except when it's seen as something separate from our relationships. If you think you might be an exception to this, it might be a useful exercise to spend a few moments reflecting on your experience of being fully yourself, that is, fully connected to yourself. Then think about how easy it is to do this in an intimate relationship, in any kind of relationship.

There is a lot of confusion about what this actually means. One version of being fully yourself is that you are able to do and say whatever spontaneously occurs to you without caring what those around you think or feel about it. Another version is where you may feel free to be fully yourself when you are alone or communing with nature but not with other people, especially not with your intimate partner.

Another sub-category of the latter pattern is when you can be fully yourself with a certain group of your friends but not with your intimate partner (often that partner will have a problem with those friends, which you will doubtless experience as yet another attempt to control you).[1] All of these versions of being and expressing ourselves fully, and there may well be other variations that I haven't mentioned, involve disconnection and distance. What I'm talking about is being able to be fully yourself – true to yourself is another way of expressing this – *and* in contact with another human being at the same time. This isn't easy. The reality is that most of us are subtly (sometimes not so subtly!) different, or we express ourselves differently, according to who we're with. That's not the point. Different relationships call forth different aspects of me, and this is entirely appropriate, especially since they are just that – aspects of *me*. I have a problem, though, if I can't be fully connected to myself and to my intimate partner at the same time, especially when making love. Paradoxically, the solution is to let go of any idea of 'identity' and just to be in the moment, in my body and in the connection with my partner.

The feeling of disconnection operates not only at the level of personal relationships but also socially and globally. At this social and ecological level, the feeling of distance is equally, if not more, damaging. If we don't feel our visceral connection to the planet that has the capacity to support and nurture us, then the concerns we may have about environmental damage remain theoretical and distant, however sincere our wish may be for our present situation to be different.

Although the therapy I've been writing about in this book is called *Sexual Grounding Therapy*, it is clear from the above reflections that the implications of the work go way beyond the physical act of sex, even though, as should be clear by now, sex and sexual energy are foundations of who we are as human beings. It is therefore not surprising that previous participants in SGT have reported rediscovering not just their sexual selves but a grounded sense of who they are as a whole person – mother, father, lover, friend, etc. All of the roles I've just mentioned describe relationships, and one of the strengths of SGT is that, by enabling participants to relate fully without projection, *all* of their relationships, not just their sexual relationships, are transformed.

The more we are able to connect with ourselves and feel comfortable with the self that we are, the more we will be able to express ourselves, and most importantly, our feelings in our relationships, especially our sexual relationships.

The resulting experience of fulfilment will have a transformative effect on our relationships with friends, family and the wider world.

Note

1 I'm definitely not talking about coercive control here, where one partner seeks to limit the contact the other has with their friends, but the situation where you may feel that your partner either does, or you believe they do, challenge you about certain behaviours that the friends, in your experience, find perfectly acceptable. A good example of this is where one partner has a concern about the other's drinking.

Appendix: Further information and useful links

Information on Sexual Grounding courses

General: www.sexualgrounding.com
France: www.trisoul.fr
Germany: www.sexualgrounding.de
Netherlands: www.sexualgrounding.nl
Mexico: www.arraigosexual.com
Russia: www.sgt-project.ru
UK, Ireland and the Channel Islands: www.psychosexualtherapycentre.co.uk/sexual-grounding.html

For all other countries, visit the general website listed above.

Other sources of information

Pelvic-Heart Integration: www.pelvic-heart-integration.eu
Sexological Bodywork: www.sexologicalbodywork.co.uk
Tantra (Diana Richardson): www.loveforcouples.com
Sex Coaching: www.lucyrowett.com
To contact the author: www.geoff-lamb-psychotherapist.com

Index

For Product Safety Concerns and Information please contact our EU
representative GPSR@taylorandfrancis.com
Taylor & Francis Verlag GmbH, Kaufingerstraße 24, 80331 München, Germany